HEART DISEASE COOKBOOK

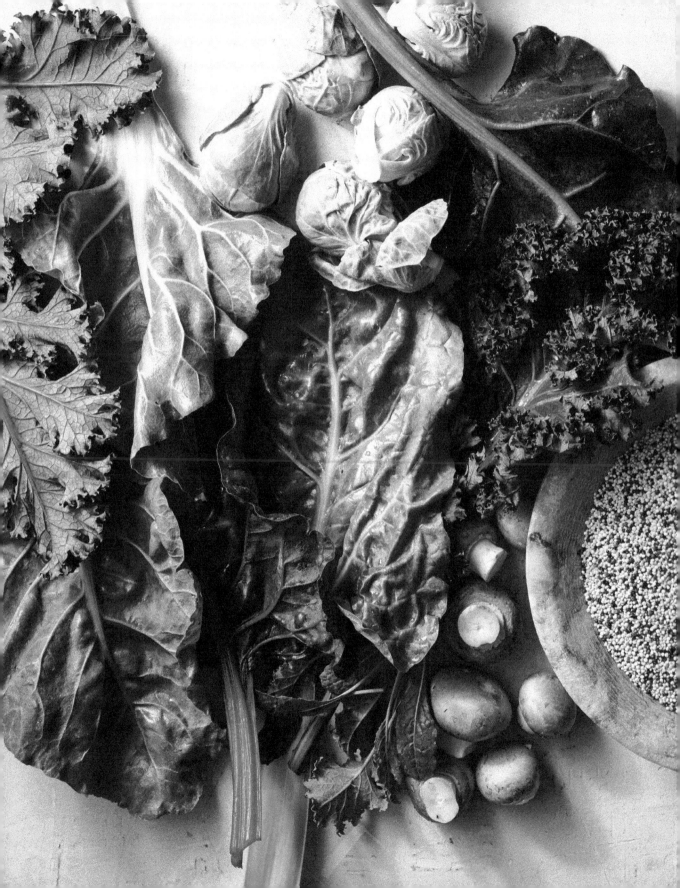

Heart Disease
COOKBOOK

EASY PLANT-BASED, HEART-HEALTHY RECIPES

KATIE REINES, MS, RD

Photography by Marija Vidal

**ROCKRIDGE
PRESS**

For general information on our other products and services or to obtain technical support, please contact our Customer Care Department within the United States at (866) 744-2665, or outside the United States at (510) 253-0500.

Rockridge Press publishes its books in a variety of electronic and print formats. Some content that appears in print may not be available in electronic books, and vice versa.

Interior and Cover Designer: Eric Pratt
Art Producer: Meg Baggott
Editor: Rachelle Cihonski
Production Manager: Martin Worthington
Production Editor: Melissa Edeburn

Photography © 2021 Marija Vidal. Food styling by Elisabet der Nederlanden.
Author photo courtesy of Ellen Tran.

ISBN: Print 978-1-64876-859-0 | eBook 978-1-64876-860-6

R1

To my incredibly supportive and open-minded
parents, Iris and Eric. Thank you for always
being there for me—even from across
the country—for practicing the recipes in this
book in their early stages, and for providing
me the sweet gift of peace through your own
transition toward plant-based eating.

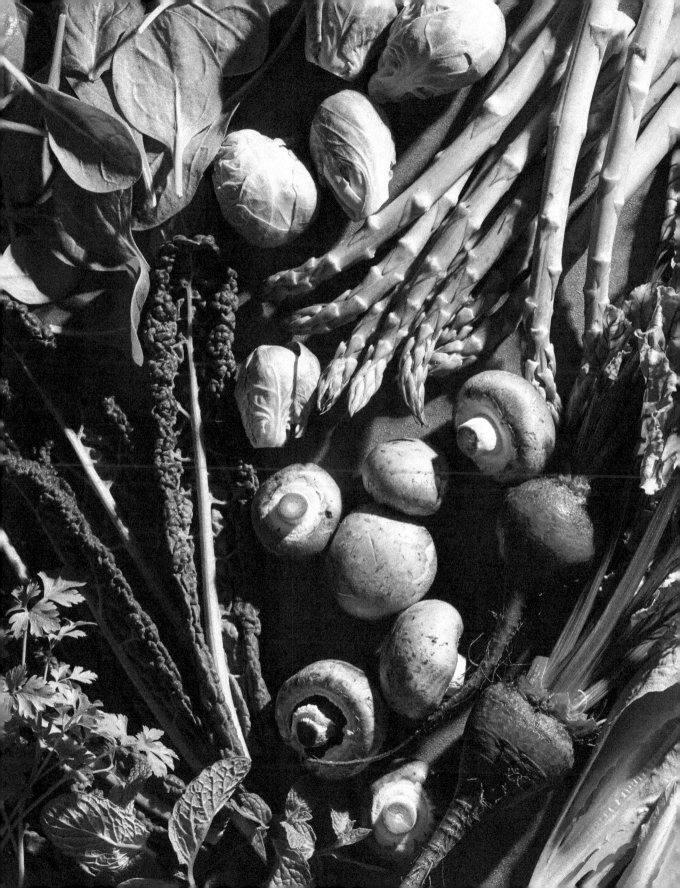

Contents

Introduction

I thought it would be impossible to help my busy client, we'll call him John, lower his cholesterol and ultimately reverse his heart disease. Not because he had an underlying genetic condition. He simply didn't want to cook. He didn't own any cooking equipment and wasn't about to get into the kitchen anytime soon.

We worked together to create a meal plan that empowered him to eat out at convenient places and still eat for heart health. He also agreed to set aside 15 minutes per week to prepare seven jars of Chia-Oat Pudding (page 29) to eat daily and took my advice on what to order for takeout. And while John may have been eating in his car, he did it! Within six weeks, his cholesterol and triglyceride levels dropped, and he got off his medications. Today, he is an inspired plant-based king in the kitchen.

As a registered dietitian with a master's degree in human nutrition, I'm here to tell you that cholesterol-related heart disease reversal doesn't have to be complicated. My dad was actually the one who told me that simple lifestyle changes were more effective than medications when it comes to heart health. My 70-year-old father is a medical doctor with a genetic predisposition to unfavorable cholesterol and triglyceride counts. Even with plenty of risk factors, he stopped taking cholesterol-lowering statins. Why?

Blood pressure– and cholesterol-lowering medications have been shown to reduce risk of cardiovascular disease by only 20 to 30 percent. On the other hand, healthy lifestyle choices like a balanced plant-based diet, consistent moderate exercise, and not smoking have been shown to reduce risk by 92 percent. However, while a no-pills approach worked for my father, it's important to check with your doctor before you stop taking any medication. Some people have a genetic condition that requires medication in addition to lifestyle changes.

Unfortunately, people often think the true cure is to pop a pill, even though the true cure might be as simple as a bowl of oatmeal. That's why this book goes the extra mile to make sure a transition to plant-based eating is realistic, enjoyable, and effective. The recipes rely on simple, wholesome, affordable ingredients, and almost all of them meet one or more of the following easy criteria: They can be on the table in 30 minutes or less, use no more than five ingredients, or require only one pot. The recipes contain no added salt, and use of added sweeteners or oil is minimal.

The evidence-based principles in this book will, without a doubt, help you on your way to a healthier heart and body, and they will bring you relief in the knowledge that eating healthy food can be fun, easy, and delicious.

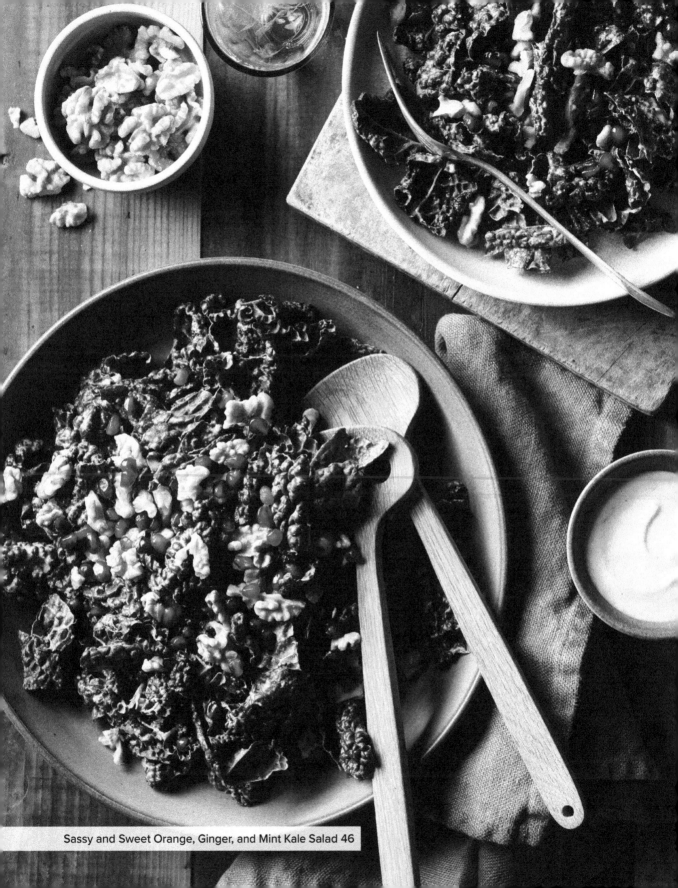

Sassy and Sweet Orange, Ginger, and Mint Kale Salad 46

1

Plant-Based, Heart-Healthy Eating Made Easy

Welcome to the plant-based diet! This book will help make your transition to a heart-healthy plant-based diet simple, straightforward, and delicious. You've already done the hard part—deciding to take a plant-based approach to your health and eating—and this book will help make the rest as smooth as possible. But first, let's start with the basics: What is a plant-based diet, and why does it work when it comes to your heart (and overall) health?

Heal Your Heart with Plants

Whether you've recently been diagnosed with heart disease, have had heart disease for years, or you are simply looking to take preventive steps, making small changes can have a monumental impact that can ensure a long and healthy life. And while going over the results of blood tests with your doctor can be overwhelming, a lot can be done to improve your numbers without spending hours in the kitchen, torturing yourself at the gym, or giving up foods you love.

There is one diet that has been proven to significantly improve heart disease and that is a plant-based diet. Why is a plant-based diet so effective? For optimal heart health, the body needs fiber, healthy fats, antioxidants, and phytochemicals, all of which are almost exclusively found in plant foods. Also, plants in their whole form contain no cholesterol, questionable additives, or trans fats. Plants are also generally low in sodium, saturated fat, and overall calories, and therefore contribute not only to heart health but also to overall well-being. The beneficial effects of a plant-based diet on heart health, blood sugars, and weight can be achieved without restricting calories.

Long-term studies and randomized controlled trials show that a plant-centric plate is superior to other options. It has been predicted that if everyone ate about 800 grams of fruits and vegetables per day (8 to 10 servings), 7.8 million premature deaths would be prevented worldwide every year.

Of course, change is not always easy. It requires rearranging priorities and trying new things. I've been there. Don't give up! You are gaining knowledge and skills on which your life depends.

What Does Eating a Plant-Based Diet Mean?

Everyone knows that a vegan diet is plant based, but eating "vegan" does not directly equate to "healthy." Therefore, this book presents a plant-based diet that emphasizes whole foods, meaning foods that are minimally processed and as close as possible to their original form: vegetables, fruits, whole grains, beans, legumes, nuts, and seeds. The diet eschews foods that are fried or that contain added sugars and preservatives. (And of course, it includes no animal products like meat, seafood, or dairy.)

But if you think a healthy plant-based diet is bland, think again. Once you remove added fat, salt, and sugar, you will be able to taste the actual flavors of whole plant foods. And you will begin to appreciate the explosions of flavor you can get from fresh herbs and spices.

That said, it is okay to use salt, oil, and sugar *very sparingly*. The recipes in this book do not call for added salt, but some do call for minimal amounts of added sweetener or oil. Both can be swapped out or left out.

If you do choose to use salt sparingly, I recommend you use iodized salt. As its name implies, iodized salt is a good source of iodine, a micronutrient important for thyroid health, hormone balance, and metabolism. If you are using oil, I recommend choosing avocado oil because it has a high smoke point and mild flavor. Olive oil is a good option, too, but be sure it is a high-quality extra-virgin variety. Limit oil whenever possible by sautéing with water, low-sodium vegetable broth, coconut aminos, or reduced-sodium soy sauce. For baked goods, try replacing half of the oil with unsweetened applesauce.

The Heart of the Plant-Based Diet

Before you go piling your plate sky high with popcorn and potatoes, let's go over the principles of a plant-based diet. Popcorn and potatoes are minimally processed foods and are fantastic to include in a plant-based diet, but you'll need to eat a variety of plant-based whole foods to get all the essential nutrients your body needs.

The five groups of foods you'll want to include in your diet are vegetables, fruits, whole grains, beans, and nuts and seeds. The first four groups are the core of the plant-based diet: Minimally processed vegetables, fruits, whole grains, and beans are full of sustainably energizing complex carbohydrates, microbiome-feasting fiber, anti-inflammatory and immune-boosting antioxidants, protein, and vitamins and minerals. These foods are generally low in calories. The fifth food group is just as important as the core four, but because nuts and seeds are calorie dense with most of their calories coming from fat, they need to be eaten in relatively small servings.

The three macronutrients—carbohydrates, protein, and fat—provide calories for us to use for energy. Fat is 9 calories per gram; carbohydrates and protein are only 4 calories per gram. The four core food groups are composed mostly of carbohydrates and protein; the last food group, nuts and seeds, is composed mostly of fat. Although essential to a healthy balanced diet, calorie-dense fat is best consumed in small servings.

To help balance your meals, make sure your plate is made up of 25 percent vegetables, 25 percent fruit, 25 percent whole grains, and 25 percent legumes. Include 1 to 4 tablespoons of nuts or seeds or ¼ avocado. Aim for a wide variety of textures, flavors, and colors.

Vegetables: Aim to eat a variety of different colored vegetables every day, multiple times a day. Be sure to include both raw and cooked vegetables in your diet to maximize nutrient intake.

Fruits: Eat a wide variety of fruits regularly but aim to include berries daily. Berries are high in antioxidants and fiber and low in sugar compared with other fruits. When it comes to blood sugar control and overall weight maintenance, the higher the water content of the fruit, the better. (Think watermelon and grapefruit.) Avocados, though technically a fruit, are mostly fat. They should be consumed in smaller portions than other fruits.

Whole grains: Whole grains include rice, quinoa, oats, and grain products made from 100-percent whole-grain flour like whole-wheat pasta. Aim for at least half of the grains you eat to be intact whole grains. For example, eat cooked quinoa (an intact whole grain) more often than tortillas made from quinoa flour (a refined grain product). Quinoa that has been processed into a flour may not have as much fiber or nutritional benefit as the "intact whole grain" quinoa. I recommend rinsing whole grains before cooking them and, if possible, soaking them for at least 8 hours or overnight for increased nutrient availability. When choosing grain products like bread, pasta, and cereal, look for the words "100-percent whole-grain" on the label, and make sure the first ingredient listed is "whole grain." If you are gluten intolerant or sensitive to grains, try substituting starchy vegetables such as potatoes or winter squash.

Legumes: Legumes such as beans, lentils, and peas are technically vegetables, but they are a tad higher in calories and protein than most other vegetables. In a plant-based diet, legumes have the honor of their own important and distinct food group. I recommend consuming 1 to 3 servings per day. If purchasing dried beans, be sure to sufficiently cook them. Undercooked beans may cause gas and stomachaches. I recommend soaking all legumes for at least 8 hours before cooking.

The soaking releases enzyme inhibitors and antinutrients that may prevent absorption of nutrients and cause indigestion. If not cooking beans from scratch, be sure to choose no-salt-added canned beans.

Nuts and seeds: Consume 1 to 4 tablespoons of high omega-3 hemp seeds, soaked chia seeds, ground flaxseed, or walnuts per meal as well as 1 to 4 tablespoons of other unsalted nuts, seeds, and nut or seed butters. These nuts and seeds will help ensure essential fatty acid intake, absorption of important fat-soluble vitamins, and production of hormones, as well as skin, eye, brain, and heart health. Without essential fats, triglycerides skyrocket, increasing inflammation and exacerbating heart disease.

FAQ: What to Know about Eating a Heart-Healthy, Plant-Based Diet

When it comes to plant-based eating, a few questions typically arise.

Q: Will a plant-based diet help with diabetes and high blood pressure?

A: Yes, a whole-foods, plant-based diet will assist your efforts to control those comorbidities.

Q: Is the diet safe if I am on medications, recovering from cardiac surgery, or both?

A: If you will be significantly shifting your diet by following the recipes in this book, consult with your doctor first. If the diet is approved, keep your doctor informed of your progress; doses of medications that help control your blood pressure, blood sugar, and cholesterol may need to be decreased within just a week. Keep in mind that your medication may have food and nutrient interactions. For example, if you are taking a statin medication, eating grapefruit will make that medication ineffective. If you are taking warfarin or other blood-thinning medication, talk with your doctor about whether you should avoid foods high in vitamin K, such as kale and broccoli, which can alter the medication's effectiveness.

If you are recovering from cardiac surgery, a plant-based diet filled with minimally processed food can be extremely helpful and set you on course for a healthier future.

Q: Can I drink coffee and alcohol?

A: How your body processes caffeine is unique to your genetic makeup. In general, I recommend keeping your coffee intake under 2 plain cups per day and consuming them before 11 a.m. Too much caffeine may exacerbate heart issues and drinking it too late in the day may disturb sleep.

When it comes to alcohol, less is better. If you must drink, maximum recommendations are one drink per day for women and two drinks per day for men. One drink is equivalent to 5 ounces of wine, 12 ounces of beer, or 1½ ounces of hard liquor. I recommend dry red wines like cabernet sauvignon or pinot noir because they contain heart-healthy antioxidants and are lower in sugar and calories than sweeter red wines.

Q: What's wrong with salt and oil?

A: It makes sense that a diet low in salt is necessary for heart health because sodium increases water retention, therefore increasing blood volume, which forces the heart to work harder. Research has shown that reducing dietary salt intake by as little as ½ teaspoon a day significantly improves endothelial function (the function of the lining of blood vessels), thus controlling vascular relaxation, contraction, and blood clotting.

Although plant-based oils are more health-promoting than fats from animal products, they still contain about 120 calories per tablespoon. Moreover, not all oils are created equal. Intake of low-quality oils or oils that have been heated past their smoke point could exacerbate heart disease issues and increase risk.

Q: Is it okay to eat faux meat on a plant-based diet?

A: If you're accustomed to eating animal products and are having strong cravings for those flavors, incorporating small portions of plant-based meat alternatives is absolutely fine as you transition to a plant-based diet. It's much better than turning away from a plant-based diet because it seems unsustainable.

Q: What, if any, supplements do I need to take?

A: I recommend three supplements: vitamin B_{12}, vitamin D_3, and an algae-derived DHA/EPA supplement. Always consult with your doctor before adding supplements to your diet.

Your Plant-Based Kitchen

This section covers the basic ingredients and tools you will need to make your plant-based diet sustainable, delicious, and fun. You will see these ingredients throughout the recipes in this book.

Fresh and Frozen Necessities

Fresh herbs, garlic, and ginger: Herbs, garlic, and ginger provide the flavor punch needed to make meals truly special without added salt. I always have fresh parsley or cilantro in the refrigerator.

Fruits, fresh or frozen: Purchase enough fresh fruit to have at least one daily serving, such as ½ cup of berries or 1 orange. Blueberries are one of the most antioxidant-rich foods, and I recommend that you consume them daily. Purchasing them frozen is a good idea because they are picked ripe and in season before being frozen, making them high in nutrients. Frozen blueberries are cheaper than fresh blueberries and will keep longer, too.

Leafy greens, fresh or frozen: Keep a variety of leafy greens, such as spinach, kale, and collard greens, on hand at all times. They are high in essential micronutrients. In fact, 1 cup of steamed collard greens has as much calcium as a glass of milk. If you're worried the fresh greens will go bad before you can use them, wash them, put them in an airtight container, and store them in the freezer. Later, you can sauté them or use them in soups or smoothies.

Lemons and limes, fresh: These popular citrus staples provide vitamin C, which helps to convert non–heme iron from plants into the bioavailable heme iron form. Squeeze some lemon or lime juice over your meals to increase iron absorption and for a bright flavor boost.

Potatoes, fresh: I recommend choosing potatoes that are full of color; the more color, the more antioxidants! Sweet potatoes come in many colors and varieties, such as sweet orange yams and Okinawan purple potatoes. My favorite is the Japanese Murasaki sweet potato. That said, don't ignore the white russet potato; it is low in fat and an incredible source of the important electrolyte, potassium. Also, all potatoes are fantastic complex carbohydrates, providing fiber and resistant starches that may benefit gut health.

Vegetables, fresh or frozen: Include vegetables in meals as often as you can. Mushrooms and onions are great to have on hand for adding meaty texture, salt-free flavor, beneficial nutrients, and immune-boosting properties. Peas and corn provide an array of complementary amino acids that combine to form a complete protein, and they are full of complex carbohydrates for lasting energy. Freezing does not alter texture and taste.

Pantry Essentials

Cacao powder: Want that decadent chocolate flavor without all the added sugar and fat? Add cacao powder to smoothies, oatmeal, yogurt parfaits, or chia pudding. Cacao powder is slightly less processed than cocoa powder; however, both work well for the recipes in this book.

Canned beans and legumes: Be sure to purchase canned items that are labeled "no-salt-added," "low-sodium," or "reduced-sodium" and have less than 300mg of sodium per serving. Canned beans are an efficient and convenient way to keep cooked beans on hand.

Dried fruit: Unsweetened raisins, dried figs, and pitted dates can add texture to any meal. They provide potassium, fiber, and antioxidants. Their super-sweet flavor makes them a good substitute for sugar.

Dried herbs and spices: A salt-free diet can be jazzed up with herbs and spices. I always have curry powder, red pepper flakes, an array of dried herbs, plus garlic, onion, and ginger powders in the cupboard. Some herbs and seasonings may provide medicinal benefits. For example, research has shown a 50 percent improvement in artery function with ingestion of just ¼ teaspoon of garlic powder per day.

Nuts and seeds and their butters: Keep walnuts, chia seeds, hemp seeds, and flaxseed in the refrigerator. Other nuts and seeds to stock up on include raw pumpkin seeds, sunflower seeds, almonds (plus almond flour), Brazil nuts, cashews, pistachios, and pecans. Nut and seed butters are another great source of healthy fats and there are a variety of options, such as almond, peanut, sunflower seed, and tahini (sesame seed) butters. Look at the ingredients label and do not purchase products with added oil, especially fully or partially hydrogenated oil, added salt, or added sugar.

Oats, rice, quinoa, millet, and buckwheat: Rolled oats are a staple on the plant-based diet because they are so versatile. (Look for those labeled gluten-free, if needed.) Blend them up into oat flour (see the tip in the Pumpkin Spice Apple-Cinnamon Pancakes recipe, page 38) to make pancakes or baked goods, use them as a base for granola or energy bars, or make a pot of porridge for breakfast. Other grains to have on hand include rice, quinoa, millet, and buckwheat.

Pasta: Stock up on whole-grain varieties, bean-based varieties, or both. You can also find pastas made with rice and quinoa and with gluten-free flours.

Vegetable broth: Be sure to choose low-sodium vegetable broth and refrigerate it after opening it. Even better, make your own (page 142) so you have absolute control over the ingredients.

Whole-grain bread, tortillas, flour, granola, and cereals: Whole-grain bread, tortillas, and whole-wheat or gluten-free all-purpose flour are all great to have stocked in your pantry. Choose whole-grain options that have little to no added sugar or oil. When purchasing cereals and granola, look for those with little to no added sugar and with 20 percent or more of the total carbohydrate grams coming from fiber.

Cooking Tools and Equipment

Cutting board: Get at least one large or a few medium and small sizes.

Food processor: If you buy only one blending appliance, I would recommend getting the blender. But a food processor can also play an important role in the kitchen. Food processors are better at blending hard and dry ingredients, whereas blenders are better with soft and wet ingredients. Invest in a food processor that has both a grating attachment and an S-shaped blade.

High-powered blender: Pulverizing whole-food ingredients, like whole avocados or nuts, requires a high-powered blender like a Vitamix.

Large (3- to 4-quart) pot: I recommend using 100-percent ceramic, cast iron, or stainless steel and avoiding Teflon, aluminum, and copper.

Large (10- to 12-inch) skillet: I recommend using 100-percent ceramic, cast iron, or stainless steel and avoiding Teflon, aluminum, and copper.

Measuring cups and spoons: Have clear measuring cups for measuring liquids and a graduated set of scoop-style measuring cups for measuring dry ingredients.

Mixing bowls: Get a range of sizes, including small ones for mixing seasonings. Get two large bowls for mixing wet and dry ingredients separately in baking recipes.

Sharp knives: One large chef's knife, one serrated bread knife, and one small paring knife should suffice.

Sheet pan: A large rimmed baking sheet is great for roasting vegetables and making baked goods.

Sieve: A large fine-mesh sieve is needed to rinse small grains like quinoa and to drain cooked pasta.

Silicone baking mat: Instead of continuing to purchase parchment paper, save a trip to the store and invest in a nonstick, food-grade, reusable silicone baking mat.

Plant-Based Heart Heroes to Love (and Buy in Bulk)

A plant-based diet will introduce you to all the delicious and healthy ingredients on the shelves of your local grocery store. Although you may not have heard of some of the ingredients used in this book's recipes, I assure you that they are not uncommon. Below, you'll discover where to find them and why they are plant-based diet rock stars.

Apple cider vinegar: Adding acid to meals with vinegar or lemon is a great way to add flavor without salt. Plus, consuming apple cider vinegar (ACV) may improve blood glucose control and reduce blood triglycerides, cholesterol, and blood pressure. You can find ACV in the condiment or baking aisle.

Hemp seeds (or hemp hearts), chia seeds, and flaxseed (or flax meal): These seeds are high in heart-healthy omega-3 fatty acids as well as in important antioxidants and fibers that have been shown to improve heart health. Eat chia seeds after they have been soaked or ground and flaxseed after they have been ground. You can find them in the nuts and seeds aisle of most grocery stores. Keep seeds high in omega-3s like hemp, chia, and flaxseed in the refrigerator to maintain their freshness.

Miso: Miso is a savory paste typically made from fermented soybeans, although it may also be made from other beans or grains. Purchase white miso (either sweet or mellow)—the dark red varieties are higher in sodium—from your local grocery store or Asian market. Miso contains beneficial probiotic bacteria that can be great for gut health if kept under boiling temperatures.

Nutritional yeast: This deactivated yeast grown on, and then harvested from, molasses is then fortified with B vitamins. It's not related to the yeast used for baking. It can be found at most grocery stores. Nutritional yeast has a rich umami flavor characteristic of cheese.

Plant-based milks: In the refrigerated section of your grocery store, you'll find many plant-based milks, including oat milk, almond milk, and soy milk. Be sure to purchase one that is unsweetened and fortified with nutrients like calcium, vitamin D_3, and vitamin B_{12}. Canned coconut milk is another plant-based milk option.

Sea vegetables: Reducing your salt intake is a great way to reduce blood pressure and improve heart health; however, the thyroid (a gland in your neck that controls hormonal function) needs iodine. That's where sea vegetables come in. You may be familiar with one of them—nori, the traditional sushi wrap. Other sea vegetables include dulse, arame, kombu, and wakame. Some come in a crushed form, available at grocery and natural foods stores in shakers similar to saltshakers.

Stevia leaf extract: Stevia is a plant that is sweeter than sugar yet does not contribute calories or cause blood glucose spikes. In recipes, I replace ¼ cup of maple syrup with 32 drops of stevia extract. Find it in the baking aisle of your local grocery store.

Tamari and coconut aminos: Tamari is a soy sauce alternative that is wheat and gluten free and that provides umami flavor. Be sure to purchase the reduced-sodium variety. Coconut aminos also provide umami flavor and are wheat and gluten free. Made from the fermented sap of coconut palm, they are the lowest-sodium alternative to soy sauce.

Tofu, tempeh, and seitan: Tofu is a soy product full of protein and protective compounds called isoflavones. Tofu soaks up flavor in sauces and spices. It ranges in texture from silken to extra firm and can be made super firm and crispy with pressing, baking, or freezing. Like tofu, tempeh is a fermented soy product; however, it is made from fermented whole beans instead of soy milk, so it has a chunkier texture. Seitan is a chewy meat alternative made from vital wheat gluten. Tempeh and seitan are both great at soaking up flavors and work well in lots of recipes in place of chicken, pork, or beef. You can purchase these products in the refrigerated section of most grocery stores.

Meal Planning How-To

One of the easiest ways to transition to and stick to a plant-based diet is to learn how to meal plan and prep. If you want to save money, dial in your nutrition, and have fun in the kitchen, you first need to ensure that your meals are balanced, delicious, easy to make, and budget friendly. Below are some helpful steps for getting started.

Calculate your budget: Here's a formula to figure out your grocery budget: *$X spent on groceries per month / Y visits to the grocery store per month = $X per grocery store visit.* For example, if I want to limit my grocery store spending to about $300 per month, and I go grocery shopping once a week, I would calculate $300 / 4 visits per month = $75 per grocery store visit.

Remember FIFO—first in, first out: It can be tempting to purchase lots of new food when you're excited about trying new recipes, but be sure to take inventory and incorporate whatever ingredients you've already got in your refrigerator, freezer, and cupboards into your meal plan first.

Master menu planning: Create a blank menu chart and begin to fill in meals that are as simple as possible. Use the ingredients you already have, keep closely to what you know and like, and make just a few tweaks, trying just three to five new plant-based foods or products per week. Include indulgences, in moderation.

Make a grocery list: Go through the recipes you'd like to try this week and make a list of the ingredients and amounts that you need. Be as specific as possible to avoid overspending and food waste. For example, note exactly how many onions you will need as opposed to simply listing "onions."

A Sample Menu

Use the weekly meal plan below to get a clear picture of what a healthy, balanced, plant-based meal plan could look like using recipes in this book. This meal plan is designed for one person. I recommend choosing no more than a handful of recipes to make in a given week and leaning heavily on at-hand ingredients and leftovers to keep both cost and active time in the kitchen as low as possible.

	BREAKFAST	LUNCH	DINNER	SNACKS AND DESSERT
SUNDAY	Peanut Butter Power Smoothie (page 26)	Buffalo Cauliflower Macaroni (page 74)	Spaghetti Squash Marinara (page 92)	1 apple, 1 to 2 tablespoons peanut butter
MONDAY	Peaches and Cream Protein Oatmeal (page 31)	Sassy and Sweet Orange, Ginger, and Mint Kale Salad (page 46), Simple Avocado and Hummus Wraps (page 57)	*Leftover* Buffalo Cauliflower Macaroni	1 cup veggies with ¼ cup Spicy Roasted Red Pepper Hummus (page 100), 1 Raw Walnut Brownie Bite (page 126)
TUESDAY	½ recipe Herbed Avocado and Chickpea Toast (page 33)	*Leftover* Sassy and Sweet Orange, Ginger, and Mint Kale Salad, *Leftover* Simple Avocado and Hummus Wraps	*Leftover* Spaghetti Squash Marinara	1 cup veggies with ¼ cup *Leftover* Spicy Roasted Red Pepper Hummus, 1 *Leftover* Raw Walnut Brownie Bite
WEDNESDAY	Peanut Butter Power Smoothie (page 26)	Hawaiian Pizzas (page 88)	*Leftover* Sassy and Sweet Orange, Ginger, and Mint Kale Salad, Simple Avocado and Hummus Wraps (page 57)	1 cup veggies with ¼ cup *Leftover* Spicy Roasted Red Pepper Hummus, 1 *Leftover* Raw Walnut Brownie Bite

	BREAKFAST	LUNCH	DINNER	SNACKS AND DESSERT
THURSDAY	*Leftover* Peaches and Cream Oatmeal	*Leftover* Sassy and Sweet Orange, Ginger, and Mint Kale Salad, *Leftover* Simple Avocado and Hummus Wraps	*Leftover* Spaghetti Squash Marinara	1 apple, 1 to 2 tablespoons peanut butter
FRIDAY	½ recipe Herbed Avocado and Chickpea Toast (page 33)	*Leftover* Hawaiian Pizzas	*Leftover* Buffalo Cauliflower Macaroni	1 cup veggies with ¼ cup *Leftover* Spicy Roasted Red Pepper Hummus, 1 *Leftover* Raw Walnut Brownie Bite
SATURDAY	Chia-Oat Pudding (page 29)	*Leftover* Hawaiian Pizzas	*Leftover* Spaghetti Squash Marinara	1 cup veggies with ¼ cup *Leftover* Spicy Roasted Red Pepper Hummus, 1 *Leftover* Raw Walnut Brownie Bite

Shopping Smarts

Don't panic if you push your budget on the first trip. The first few grocery trips could surpass your budget. If you have little to no FIFO ingredients to use, remember that many of these items will probably last a couple of weeks. Planning ahead, purchasing whole plant foods and simple products, buying in bulk, and avoiding convenience foods will save you a lot of money down the road.

Divide your shopping list into sections. Produce, grocery, baking, bulk, refrigerated, frozen—categorize each ingredient on your list to speed up shopping and avoid getting distracted by items not on your list.

Go for store brands first. Store-brand items are usually the same quality as big-brand items, yet cheaper. Remember that just because something is on sale does not mean you need to get it. Stick to your list.

Buy in bulk. Purchasing nuts, seeds, grains, and beans from bulk bins is a great way to save money and decrease waste. Some grocery stores allow you to bring your own bags or jars; weigh them ahead of time with the help of a cashier or grocery clerk, and fill them up.

Always read the labels of canned, boxed, or jarred items. Purchase foods that are as minimally processed as possible. For grain products, the first ingredient on the ingredient list should be "whole grain." Always read ingredient labels to avoid products with added sugar, processed oils, and salt. Be sure that canned or boxed items, like canned beans or vegetable broth, and premade ingredients, like hummus, salsa, or BBQ sauce, are labeled "low-sodium," "no sodium," or "no-salt-added" or have less than 300mg of sodium per serving.

Skip packaged snacks and beverages. Instead of processed packaged convenience foods, snack on whole foods like fruit, sliced veggies, nuts, and seeds. And increase your intake of water.

Don't go shopping on an empty stomach! If you go grocery shopping hungry, you're likely to get more than you need. Have a snack before you go so you can stay calm and stick to your list.

Cooking Tips for Simple and Flavorful Meals

Use the water-sauté method. Instead of using oil to sauté vegetables, try using low-sodium vegetable broth, water with miso, coconut aminos, reduced-sodium tamari or soy sauce, or just plain water. Heat the pan over medium-high heat, add about 3 tablespoons of water, then add the vegetables. Stir frequently and keep adding water, about 2 tablespoons at a time, as needed.

Opt for oil-free baking. Use a reusable silicone baking mat or parchment paper to prevent sticking instead of greasing pans. In place of oil for baked goods, use mashed avocado, banana, or sweet potato, nut or seed butters, canned pumpkin, or applesauce. To roast vegetables, coat them with tahini or balsamic vinegar instead of oil.

Add contrast. The best meals have texture or temperature contrasts or both. Add crunch to the smooth, spice to the sweet, cold to the heat, dense to the light, and moist to the dry. Next time you prepare a meal, think: What can I do to heighten contrast? I usually garnish soups and salads with seeds and raisins to create contrast.

Get saucy. Keep experimenting until you have a few salt-, oil-, and sugar-free sauces that you know and love. For me, adding a touch of ginger mixed with lemon and peanut butter or a little hot sauce goes a long way. Even just lemon juice or simple Lemon-Tahini Dressing (page 141) is often exactly what a dish needs to make it complete.

Natural spice is nice. Jalapeño, ginger, garlic, red pepper flakes, salt-free chili powder, curry powder, and cayenne pepper add flavor with zero added salt. A little goes a long way.

Lean on herbs and seasonings. Don't let those flavorful dried herbs in the cupboard go to waste. It takes time to get to know your herb, seasoning, and flavor profile preferences. Experiment with different herbs instead of salt. You can also find prepackaged salt-free seasoning blends, such as Italian seasoning and taco seasoning.

Easing into Your New Plant-Based Diet

If the switch to a plant-based diet feels overwhelming, imagine the most positive result. The following tips will help you to keep moving forward.

I've never cooked before—where do I start? Incorporate one to three new plant-based foods or recipes into your rotation each week. Don't drastically change your meals yet; just add one plant food to your meals at a time.

Grocery shopping overwhelms me. What do I do? Order online for pickup or delivery. Also, know that it takes time to learn where things are located in each grocery store. Don't be embarrassed to ask for help.

What if I really don't have time to cook? Look up healthy options available online or at grab-and-go places near you, or get what you usually get with a side of vegetables, beans, or whole grains.

What if I want to eat out? It is okay to indulge yourself once in a while. However, if you are eating out daily or weekly, do what you can to modify what you order to be plant based and steamed, poached, or baked rather than fried. Try to keep it low in sodium, fat, and sugar and add a side of vegetables, beans, whole grains, or salad.

What do I do during the holidays? Celebrate without overdoing it and continue your routine afterward. The holidays should not be an excuse to eat too many treats for breakfast, lunch, and dinner. Pair indulgences with plenty of plants.

I ate something I shouldn't have. What now? All foods fit into a healthy, balanced, plant-based diet. There is no "wagon" to fall off. What matters are portion sizes and frequency of different food choices. So, when it comes to eating something you shouldn't have, the dose determines the poison. If you ate too much of something unhealthy, like fast food or a dessert, and are feeling uncomfortable, be sure to drink plenty of water and wait for true hunger to be present before you eat again. Though your routine should largely involve eating minimally processed plant foods, occasionally you should include the foods you crave and love to make sure a plant-based diet is sustainable for you. The important thing is to keep the portion size of those occasional indulgences small.

About the Recipes

The recipes in this book are designed to be as delicious and healthy as possible. They are completely plant based and nearly all of them meet at least one of three "easy-to-make" criteria: five or fewer ingredients (excluding water and pepper), 30 minutes or less to make, or requiring just one vessel for both preparation and cooking. The recipes offer options for substituting ingredients and varying preparation methods.

If you are new to cooking, plant-based eating, or both, the recipes may initially require some effort—but don't be discouraged. Read the recipes thoroughly a few times before starting. As you become more comfortable with plant-based cooking, the recipes will get easier. Anything new requires practice. I encourage you to stick with it—the results are worth it.

Sodium, Sugar, and Fat Content

The recipes in this book are designed to help you improve heart health through plant-based nutrition. They follow the American Heart Association's (AHA) sodium and fat guidelines with no added salt and minimal amounts of added oil and sweetener.

The AHA's recommendations are to reduce saturated and highly processed fats and to keep daily sodium intake below 1,500mg per day. Per serving, nearly all of the recipes contain less than 25g total fat and less than 7g saturated fat. The vast majority are low in sodium; most are below 350mg, and those below 140mg have the "Extra-Low Sodium" label.

In the recipes, you will often see ingredients that can be homemade or purchased. I recommend preparing the homemade versions of these ingredients, like tortillas and BBQ sauce, whenever possible to keep sodium levels low. Nutritional facts were calculated on the basis of the homemade ingredients, so keep in mind that if you opt for a store-bought alternative, the sodium level may be higher than that indicated at the bottom of the recipe.

Most of the recipes—even the desserts!—contain less than 5g of added sugar. Most contain no added sweetener. A few do include a tablespoon or two of maple syrup, for which date paste, stevia extract and water, or Truvia granulated stevia can be substituted.

Dietary Labels and Recipe Tips

To help meet your unique requirements, recipes are also labeled "Gluten-Free" when applicable. Unless you have celiac disease or are sensitive to gluten, there's no need to avoid gluten.

Most recipes include these helpful tips:

- **Make it easier**—ways to further simplify the recipe

- **Substitute it**—ingredients that may be used in place of listed ingredients

- **Flavor boost**—ideas for adding flavor

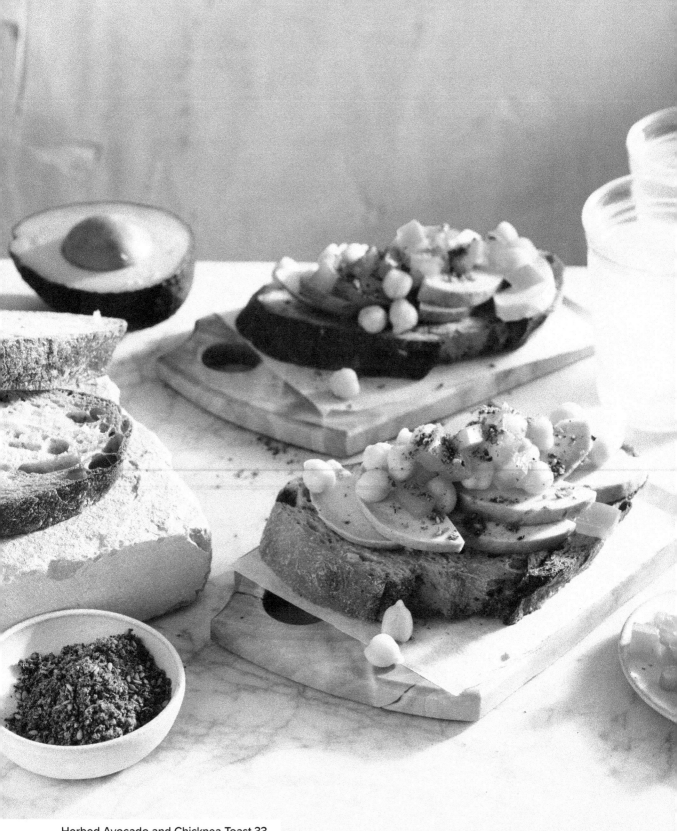

Breakfasts and Smoothies

Peanut Butter Power Smoothie

5 Ingredients or Fewer, 30 Minutes or Less, Gluten-Free, One-Pot
Serves 1 / Prep time: 5 minutes

This recipe is a favorite of my clients who are new to a plant-based diet. Flaxseed contains heart-healthy essential fats, and leafy greens are loaded with immune-boosting vitamin C and calming magnesium. When buying peanut butter, look for jars with only one ingredient on the label: dry-roasted unsalted peanuts.

2 cups spinach

1½ bananas, sliced and frozen

1 cup unsweetened vanilla plant-based milk

2 tablespoons whole or ground flaxseed

1½ tablespoons unsalted, unsweetened peanut butter

1. In a high-powered blender, combine the spinach, frozen bananas, milk, flaxseed, and peanut butter and blend until smooth.

2. Pour into a glass and enjoy immediately.

Substitute it: If you're using fresh (not frozen) bananas, add 1 cup of ice before blending. To freeze bananas, peel ripe bananas with brown spots and break into 1- to 2-inch pieces. Place the pieces in a freezer-safe container or zip-top bag, leaving space between them so they don't stick together, and freeze for at least 6 hours or overnight.

Per serving: Calories: 458; Total Fat: 25g; Saturated Fat: 3.5g; Cholesterol: 0mg; Sodium: 170mg; Carbohydrates: 55g; Fiber: 14g; Total Sugar: 25g; Added Sugar: 2g; Protein: 14g; Potassium: 1,309mg; Magnesium: 218mg; Vitamin K: 292mcg

Vibrancy Smoothie

30 Minutes or Less, Extra-Low Sodium, Gluten-Free, One-Pot
Serves 2 / Prep time: 15 minutes

After pulling an all-nighter, my roommate had three sips of this smoothie and said, "This is giving me more energy than a double shot of espresso!" With this smoothie, you, too, may discover that you are a morning person. To lower the (natural) sugar content of this smoothie, you can swap the frozen pineapple for ice. For the soy yogurt, I like Silk, Lavva, or Kite Hill brands.

2 cups packed spinach

2 cups coconut water

Juice of 1 lemon

2 bananas, fresh or frozen

1 cup frozen pineapple chunks

⅔ cup plain soy yogurt

6 tablespoons hemp seeds

1. In a high-powered blender, add the ingredients in this order: spinach, coconut water, lemon juice, bananas, pineapple, yogurt, and hemp seeds so the liquid and greens are closest to the blade.

2. Blend until smooth, pour into two glasses, and enjoy immediately.

Make it easier: Afraid your fresh spinach will go bad before you have a chance to eat it? While fresh spinach may only last about a week, frozen spinach can last much longer. Wash it and put it in a zip-top bag or a freezer-safe container to freeze for up to 1 month.

Per serving: Calories: 419; Total Fat: 17g; Saturated Fat: 2g; Cholesterol: 0mg; Sodium: 134mg; Carbohydrates: 59g; Fiber: 8g; Total Sugar: 30g; Added Sugar: 2g; Protein: 16g; Potassium: 1,617mg; Magnesium: 312mg; Vitamin K: 223mcg

Black Forest Cherry-Beet Smoothie

30 Minutes or Less, One-Pot
Serves 2 / Prep time: 15 minutes

Beets have been shown to improve oxygen utilization by 19 percent, and cherries have been shown to have incredible anti-inflammatory effects. This smoothie will help you flow through the day feeling satisfied, energized, and grounded. Use frozen banana in this smoothie, if you have it.

1½ cups unsweetened plain almond milk

3 tablespoons cacao powder

2 tablespoons hemp seeds

¼ small beet

3 bananas, fresh or frozen

¼ cup rolled oats

½ cup frozen pitted cherries

1 pitted Medjool date

1 tablespoon unsalted, unsweetened almond butter

1 teaspoon vanilla extract

1. In a high-powered blender, combine the almond milk, cacao powder, hemp seeds, beet, bananas, oats, cherries, date, almond butter, and vanilla and blend until smooth.

2. Pour into two glasses and enjoy immediately.

Flavor boost: If you don't like raw beets, use less than ¼ small beet. If you like the flavor of beets, add more next time.

Per serving: Calories: 424; Total Fat: 13g; Saturated Fat: 1g; Cholesterol: 0mg; Sodium: 145mg; Carbohydrates: 73g; Fiber: 12g; Total Sugar: 38g; Added Sugar: 0g; Protein: 11g; Potassium: 1,333mg; Magnesium: 178mg; Vitamin K: 3mcg

Chia-Oat Pudding

5 Ingredients or Fewer, 30 Minutes or Less, One-Pot
Serves 1 / Prep time: 5 minutes, plus 10 minutes to chill

Yes, this is the chia pudding that was responsible for lowering the cholesterol of one of my clients (see page viii). Line up those mason jars and make a few extra servings of this pudding so you'll have one for every day of the week. These are perfect grab-and-go breakfasts, snacks, or desserts and are full of heart disease–reversing soluble fiber, omega-3 fatty acids, and anti-inflammatory antioxidants.

¾ cup rolled oats

2 tablespoons chia seeds

½ cup frozen blueberries

1 cup unsweetened plain soy milk

1. In a small airtight container, combine the oats, chia seeds, blueberries, and soy milk and mix well. Cover and let sit in the refrigerator for at least 10 minutes before eating.

2. Serve chilled. Store leftovers in an airtight container in the refrigerator for up to 1 week.

Flavor boost: Try mixing in different fixings, like cacao powder, unsalted peanut butter, raisins, chopped raw walnuts, ground flaxseed, ground cinnamon, or vanilla extract. Also, if you're looking to gain muscle, add a scoop of your favorite plant-based protein powder and a little extra soy milk.

Per serving: Calories: 400; Total Fat: 13g; Saturated Fat: 2g; Cholesterol: 0mg; Sodium: 182mg; Carbohydrates: 61g; Fiber: 15g; Total Sugar: 9g; Added Sugar: 0g; Protein: 13g; Potassium: 510mg; Magnesium: 181mg; Vitamin K: 154mcg

Simple Serene Green Oats

5 Ingredients or Fewer, 30 Minutes or Less, Extra-Low Sodium, One-Pot
Makes 4 jars / Prep time: 10 minutes, plus 15 minutes to chill

This recipe is the perfect on-the-go option for busy people. Kids love the green color and adults love the fact that it's high in vitamins, minerals, protein, fiber, antioxidants, and healthy fats. Make it your own by mixing in whatever toppings you like.

3 cups unsweetened vanilla soy milk

1½ cups spinach

2 cups rolled oats

4 tablespoons chia seeds

4 tablespoons raisins

1. In a high-powered blender, combine the milk and spinach and blend until smooth, 30 to 60 seconds.

2. Divide the mixture evenly into four mason jars or small lidded containers. Top each container with ½ cup rolled oats, 1 tablespoon chia seeds, and 1 tablespoon raisins. Stir each container well to combine and place them in the refrigerator for at least 15 minutes or overnight to thicken.

3. Serve chilled. Store leftovers in an airtight container in the refrigerator for up to 1 week.

Per serving (1 jar): Calories: 387; Total Fat: 11g; Saturated Fat: 2g; Cholesterol: 0mg; Sodium: 105mg; Carbohydrates: 58g; Fiber: 12g; Total Sugar: 14g; Added Sugar: 0g; Protein: 15g; Potassium: 580mg; Magnesium: 141mg; Vitamin K: 120mcg

Peaches and Cream Protein Oatmeal

5 Ingredients or Fewer, 30 Minutes or Less, One-Pot
Serves 2 / Prep time: 5 minutes / Cook time: 5 minutes

This sweet, creamy oatmeal is extra satisfying because adding protein to meals is a great way to help you feel fuller longer. Protein also helps blunt blood sugar spikes and is helpful if you're looking to build or maintain muscle mass.

1 cup rolled oats

1 scoop unsweetened vanilla plant-based protein powder

1½ cups frozen sliced peaches

2 cups unsweetened vanilla soy milk, plus more as needed

½ cup unsweetened vanilla soy or almond yogurt, or homemade Fresh Walnut Yogurt (page 144)

1. In a small pot, combine the oats, protein powder, peaches, and soy milk. Heat over medium-low heat for about 5 minutes, or until the liquid is absorbed by the oats. Stir often to prevent burning. Add 2 or more additional tablespoons soy milk or water to adjust thickness as needed.

2. Transfer to two serving bowls and top each with ¼ cup yogurt. Enjoy immediately.

Flavor boost: Feel free to use whatever fruit you like instead of peaches, and top with chopped raw walnuts, hemp seeds, or Blueberry Chia Jelly (page 132) to get in those omega-3s.

Per serving: Calories: 386; Total Fat: 10g; Saturated Fat: 1g; Cholesterol: 0mg; Sodium: 287mg; Carbohydrates: 51g; Fiber: 9g; Total Sugar: 14g; Added Sugar: 2g; Protein: 27g; Potassium: 656mg; Magnesium: 123mg; Vitamin K: 3.5mcg

Cinnamon, Banana, and Beet Breakfast Balls

30 Minutes or Less, Extra-Low Sodium, One-Pot
Makes 12 breakfast balls / Prep time: 20 minutes

Are you pressed for time in the morning and need breakfast in a pinch? Make these ahead to have throughout the week! Antioxidant pigments called anthocyanins give beets, blueberries, cherries, and red cabbage their dark red/purple color. Research has shown anthocyanins to be associated with lower inflammation levels.

2 cups quick-cooking or rolled oats

2 teaspoons ground cinnamon

⅔ cup mashed banana

⅓ cup unsalted, unsweetened almond or peanut butter

2 teaspoons vanilla extract

⅔ cup grated raw beet

½ cup raw walnuts, chopped

¼ cup ground flaxseed

2 full droppers liquid stevia (optional)

1. In a large bowl, combine the oats, cinnamon, banana, almond butter, vanilla, beet, walnuts, flaxseed, and stevia (if using) and mix well. If the dough is too loose, add more oats; if it is too dry, add more mashed banana.

2. Roll into 12 balls. Store leftovers in an airtight container in the refrigerator for up to 1 week or in the freezer for up to 2 to 3 weeks.

Per serving (3 breakfast balls): Calories: 465; Total Fat: 27g; Saturated Fat: 3g; Cholesterol: 0mg; Sodium: 45mg; Carbohydrates: 51g; Fiber: 12g; Total Sugar: 9g; Added Sugar: 0g; Protein: 15g; Potassium: 660mg; Magnesium: 159mg; Vitamin K: 3mcg

Herbed Avocado and Chickpea Toast

30 Minutes or Less, One-Pot
Serves 2 / Prep time: 10 minutes / Cook time: 5 minutes

Make this breakfast staple as simple or as extravagant as you like. Just plain avocado on toast with a little garlic powder goes a long way. If you add tomato, sliced cucumber, roasted chickpeas, your favorite dried herbs (I like Italian seasoning, za'atar, or dried dill), and fresh cracked pepper, you've got yourself a white tablecloth–worthy gourmet treat.

4 slices low-sodium whole-grain bread

2 garlic cloves, halved

1 avocado, sliced

8 tablespoons no-salt-added canned chickpeas, drained and rinsed, or Spicy Roasted Chickpeas (page 98)

1 tomato, diced

2 teaspoons salt-free dried herb blend

½ teaspoon freshly ground black pepper

1. Toast the bread and rub the cut garlic evenly over each piece. (Go heavy or light, depending on your love of garlic.)

2. Spread ¼ avocado evenly on each piece of toast. Top each with 2 tablespoons chickpeas, pressing them down firmly. Dividing evenly, top with diced tomato, dried herbs, and pepper. Enjoy immediately.

Flavor boost: Instead of ¼ avocado on each slice of toast, use 1 tablespoon Herbed Chickpea Spread (page 136). Drizzle each piece with lemon juice, hot sauce, or 1 tablespoon of Lemon-Tahini Dressing (page 141) for added flavor.

Per serving: Calories: 405; Total Fat: 18g; Saturated Fat: 3g; Cholesterol: 0mg; Sodium: 305mg; Carbohydrates: 51g; Fiber: 15g; Total Sugar: 7g; Added Sugar: 0g; Protein: 14g; Potassium: 927mg; Magnesium: 104mg; Vitamin K: 34mcg

Tofu Scramble Tostadas

30 Minutes or Less, Extra-Low Sodium, Gluten-Free
Serves 4 / Prep time: 15 minutes / Cook time: 10 minutes

It is amazing what spices and nutritional yeast can do to bring flavor without any salt. These tostadas are perfect if you're looking for something savory and satisfying. And they're a good way to use whatever vegetables you have in the fridge.

1 (14-ounce) block extra-firm or firm tofu

¼ cup nutritional yeast

¼ teaspoon ground turmeric

1 teaspoon paprika

½ teaspoon garlic powder

½ teaspoon freshly ground black pepper

Juice of 1 lime, divided

¼ cup chopped red onion

¼ cup chopped mushrooms

¼ cup chopped red bell pepper

2 garlic cloves, minced

1 cup chopped kale

4 small corn tortillas

1 avocado, sliced

Salsa, sriracha, or hot sauce of choice (choose low-sodium brands), for serving

1. Wrap the tofu in a kitchen towel and press evenly and firmly to get most of the liquid out, but don't break the tofu up.

2. In a medium bowl, mash the tofu, then mix in the nutritional yeast, turmeric, paprika, garlic powder, pepper, and most of the lime juice.

3. In a nonstick skillet, water-sauté (see page 18) the onion, mushrooms, and bell pepper over medium heat for about 5 minutes, stirring frequently.

4. Add the garlic, kale, and mashed tofu mixture to the pan and mix well to combine. Cook for another 2 minutes.

5. In a separate nonstick medium skillet, heat both sides of the tortillas over medium-high heat for about 3 minutes, or until golden brown. Remove from the heat.

6. Dividing evenly, top the tortillas with tofu scramble and avocado. Add a squeeze of lime juice.

7. Serve with hot sauce(s) of choice. Store leftover tofu scramble in an airtight container in the refrigerator for up to 1 week.

Flavor boost: If you feel like your scramble needs a little salt, it's OK to add a pinch. It is a lot more beneficial to add a pinch of salt to a healthy meal like this than to give up on trying new recipes. It will take time for your taste buds to adjust to less salt, but you will get there. If you can take the heat, you can add extra flavor with minced jalapeño, red pepper flakes, or a pinch of cayenne.

Per serving: Calories: 243; Total Fat: 12g; Saturated Fat: 2g; Cholesterol: 0mg; Sodium: 33mg; Carbohydrates: 21g; Fiber: 6g; Total Sugar: 2g; Added Sugar: 0g; Protein: 17g; Potassium: 577mg; Magnesium: 74mg; Vitamin K: 32mcg

"Cheesy" Broccoli Frittata

5 Ingredients or Fewer, Extra-Low Sodium, Gluten-Free
Serves 8 / Prep time: 15 minutes / Cook time: 40 minutes

This recipe is one that must be shared with all of your friends. They are going to be impressed by how good it tastes and confused as to how just five simple ingredients come together to create a frittata with such a perfect egg-like consistency and flavor. Serve this frittata over a bed of steamed greens with fresh tomato, lime, avocado, scallion, salsa, or your favorite hot sauce. Or jazz it up with more spices, like salt-free chili powder, garlic powder, onion powder, turmeric, black pepper, or a dash of cayenne or red pepper flakes.

3 cups chopped broccoli florets

½ avocado, mashed

1½ cups unsweetened plain almond milk

1¼ cups chickpea flour

2 tablespoons nutritional yeast

1. Preheat the oven to 350°F. Line a 9-inch springform cake pan with a round of parchment paper.

2. Place the broccoli in the springform and set aside.

3. In a large bowl, vigorously whisk together the avocado and milk until smooth, about 2 minutes.

4. Add the chickpea flour and nutritional yeast and stir to combine. Pour the frittata batter into the cake pan to cover the broccoli.

5. Bake for 40 minutes, or until it begins to crack. Remove from the oven, allow to cool for at least 10 minutes, and serve warm. Store leftovers in an airtight container in the refrigerator for up to 1 week.

Substitute it: Instead of mashed avocado, try mashing ½ block of tofu or boiling ½ cup of raw Brazil nuts, pumpkin seeds, almonds, cashews, or macadamia nuts, and blending the soaked nuts or tofu with the milk for the batter. Or whisk in ¼ cup of almond butter. Experiment with using 3 cups of whatever vegetables you like in place of broccoli. I like using 1 cup of chopped asparagus, 1 cup of chopped mushrooms, and 1 cup of chopped red bell pepper. If you don't have almond milk, use another unsweetened plant-based milk, Save-the-Scraps Vegetable Stock (page 142), or just plain water.

Per serving: Calories: 110; Total Fat: 3g; Saturated Fat: 0g; Cholesterol: 0mg; Sodium: 59mg; Carbohydrates: 15g; Fiber: 4g; Total Sugar: 3g; Added Sugar: 0g; Protein: 6g; Potassium: 367mg; Magnesium: 43mg; Vitamin K: 38mcg

Pumpkin Spice Apple-Cinnamon Pancakes

30 Minutes or Less
Serves 5 / Prep time: 15 minutes / Cook time: 15 minutes

When my chef friend Josie tried these pancakes, she said the flavor was a cross between a sweet molasses cookie and a gingerbread house, and the texture was a cross between a muffin and a pancake. If you prefer thinner cakes, feel free to add more soy milk. These are also great to make ahead, freeze, and pop in the toaster when you're on the go. Sprinkle with more chopped walnuts or apples, a drizzle of maple syrup, or a dash of cinnamon before serving. Blueberry Chia Jelly (page 132) also makes a great topping.

2½ cups oat flour, store-bought or homemade (see Tip)

1 teaspoon baking soda

2 teaspoons pumpkin pie spice

⅔ cup canned unsweetened pumpkin puree

1½ cups unsweetened vanilla soy milk

¾ cup Apple-Cinnamon Sauce (page 133), plus more for topping

2 teaspoons vanilla extract

⅔ cup chopped raw walnuts

⅔ cup chopped apples

½ teaspoon avocado oil or avocado oil cooking spray

1. In a large bowl, mix together the oat flour, baking soda, and pumpkin pie spice. Set aside.

2. In a medium bowl, mix together the pumpkin puree, soy milk, apple-cinnamon sauce, and vanilla. Pour the wet ingredients into the dry ingredients and gently fold to combine. Fold in the walnuts and apples.

3. In a large skillet, heat just enough oil to prevent sticking (or mist the pan with cooking spray) over medium-low heat. Once it is hot

enough that drops of water bubble on contact, ladle ¼ cupfuls of the batter into the pan without overcrowding.

4. Cook for about 2 minutes, or until bubbles form around the edges. Flip the pancakes and cook for another 2 minutes. Repeat with the remaining batter.

5. Serve warm topped with more apple-cinnamon sauce. Store leftovers in an airtight container in the refrigerator for up to 1 week.

Make it easier: To make your own oat flour, using a high-powered blender or food processor, blend rolled or quick-cooking oats for about 1 minute or until it resembles flour, scraping down the sides as needed. You can also swap in all-purpose flour or whatever flour you prefer.

Per serving: Calories: 418; Total Fat: 19g; Saturated Fat: 2g; Cholesterol: 0mg; Sodium: 280mg; Carbohydrates: 51g; Fiber: 10g; Total Sugar: 7g; Added Sugar: 0g; Protein: 14g; Potassium: 470mg; Magnesium: 136mg; Vitamin K: 2.4mcg

Turmeric Milk French Toast

30 Minutes or Less
Serves 3 / Prep time: 10 minutes / Cook time: 15 minutes

Anti-inflammatory French toast? Yes! This recipe is inspired by the traditional beverage in India called golden milk, or turmeric milk. Turmeric provides myriad health benefits, including reducing inflammation, improving immunity, and even decreasing the risk of chronic disease. Serve these topped with chopped raw walnuts and Blueberry Chia Jelly (page 132) or Apple-Cinnamon Sauce (page 133).

2 tablespoons ground flaxseed

1 cup unsweetened vanilla soy milk

9 slices whole-grain bread

1 teaspoon vanilla extract

1½ teaspoons pumpkin pie spice

½ teaspoon ground turmeric

Pinch freshly ground black pepper

½ teaspoon avocado oil or avocado oil cooking spray

1. In a medium bowl, combine the flaxseed and milk and let it sit for at least 5 minutes, until thickened, to create a flax "egg."

2. Meanwhile, toast the bread and set aside.

3. Stir the vanilla, pumpkin pie spice, turmeric, and black pepper into the flax egg.

4. Grease a large nonstick skillet with the oil (or mist with cooking spray) to prevent sticking. Warm the skillet over medium-low heat.

5. Quickly dip each piece of bread into the spice and flax egg mixture on each side without soaking it and place a few slices in the skillet. Cook the toast for about 2 minutes on each side. It should flip easily without sticking.

6. Repeat with the remaining slices of bread and serve warm. Store leftovers in an airtight container in the refrigerator for up to 1 week.

Substitute it: Enjoy these warming spices with whatever bread you have, such as whole wheat or sourdough. For a fun option, after cooking, cut the toast into four pieces to make French toast sticks and keep in the freezer to reheat and eat throughout the week.

Per serving: Calories: 326; Total Fat: 8g; Saturated Fat: 1g; Cholesterol: 0mg; Sodium: 480mg; Carbohydrates: 49g; Fiber: 8g; Total Sugar: 8g; Added Sugar: 0g; Protein: 16g; Potassium: 396mg; Magnesium: 113mg; Vitamin K: 10mcg

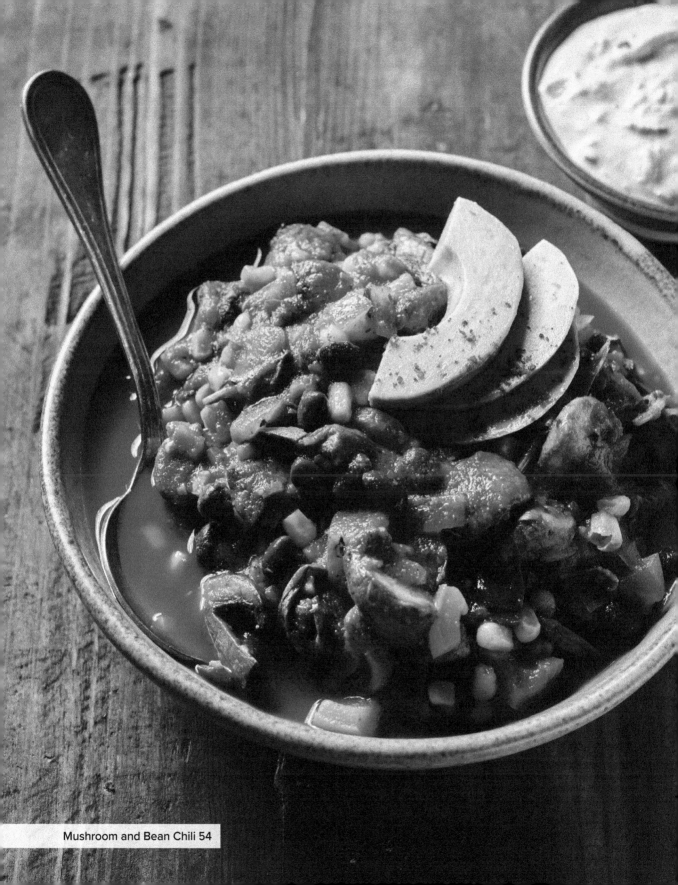

Mushroom and Bean Chili 54

Salads, Soups, and Sandwiches

Tomato and Corn Fiesta Salad

30 Minutes or Less, Extra-Low Sodium, Gluten-Free, One-Pot
Serves 4 / Prep time: 15 minutes, plus 10 minutes to chill

In the summer, when farmers' market tomatoes taste like candy, this salad is a necessity. It is fun to serve alongside rice and beans, in a burrito or taco, or as a refreshing snack. Combining avocado with jalapeño provides the perfect balance of calm and smooth with fiery and spicy.

2 cups diced tomatoes

1 cup diced zucchini

1 cup frozen corn, thawed

⅓ cup diced onion

1 avocado, cubed

Juice of 1 lemon

3 tablespoons diced jalapeño

½ teaspoon garlic powder

¼ teaspoon ground cumin

1. In a large bowl, combine the tomatoes, zucchini, corn, onion, avocado, lemon juice, jalapeño, garlic powder, and cumin. Stir well.

2. Chill for at least 10 minutes before serving. Store leftovers in an airtight container in the refrigerator for up to 3 days.

Make it easier: If you're not going to be eating this right away, keep the avocado out and add it just before serving. Avocado will turn brown after a day or two, but the other ingredients can last in the fridge for up to 1 week. To help prevent the avocado from turning brown, be sure to squeeze some lemon directly on the avocado—the vitamin C from the lemon juice acts as a powerful antioxidant to prevent oxidation or browning. This also works with other fruits that are a bit lower in vitamin C like apples and bananas.

Per serving: Calories: 128; Total Fat: 6g; Saturated Fat: 1g; Cholesterol: 0mg; Sodium: 12mg; Carbohydrates: 19g; Fiber: 5g; Total Sugar: 6g; Added Sugar: 0g; Protein: 3g; Potassium: 639mg; Magnesium: 42mg; Vitamin K: 17mcg

Quinoa-Pomegranate Holiday Salad

Extra-Low Sodium, Gluten-Free, One-Pot
Serves 4 / Prep time: 10 minutes, plus 10 minutes to chill / Cook time: 15 minutes

This is my spin on traditional tabbouleh, a Middle Eastern vegetarian salad, and is the absolute perfect dish to bring to any holiday party. It has such a variety of colors, textures, and flavors going on that every bite feels like a party in your mouth. Add fresh herbs, nuts, and fruits you like for variety.

3 cups water

1 cup quinoa, rinsed

Juice of 1 lemon

1 cup pomegranate seeds

½ cup chopped fresh parsley

½ cup chopped fresh mint

⅓ cup raw pumpkin seeds

⅓ cup raisins

1. In a medium saucepan, bring the water to a boil over high heat. Add the quinoa, reduce the heat to medium, and simmer for about 15 minutes, or until the water is absorbed and the quinoa is light and fluffy.

2. Meanwhile, in a large bowl, combine the lemon juice, pomegranate seeds, parsley, mint, pumpkin seeds, and raisins.

3. Add the cooked quinoa and refrigerate for at least 10 minutes. Serve chilled. Store leftovers in an airtight container in the refrigerator for up to 1 week.

Per serving: Calories: 312; Total Fat: 8g; Saturated Fat: 1g; Cholesterol: 0mg; Sodium: 17mg; Carbohydrates: 52g; Fiber: 7g; Total Sugar: 20g; Added Sugar: 0g; Protein: 12g; Potassium: 636mg; Magnesium: 102mg; Vitamin K: 135mcg

Sassy and Sweet Orange, Ginger, and Mint Kale Salad

30 Minutes or Less, Extra-Low Sodium, Gluten-Free, One-Pot
Serves 4 / Prep time: 20 minutes

The bright lemon, orange, and refreshing mint combined with warmth from ginger in this salad is like a rejuvenating ray of sunshine. When my roommate tried this salad, she kept saying, "You could serve this in a restaurant!" It definitely tastes gourmet yet is so simple. Save the kale stems to dip in hummus, chop up and throw in a soup, or, if you have a juicer, juice them.

8 cups stemmed and chopped kale

2 oranges, peeled

¼ cup raw cashews

¼ cup packed fresh mint leaves

2 teaspoons grated fresh ginger or ground ginger

Juice of 2 lemons

3 pitted Medjool dates

⅔ cup pomegranate seeds

⅔ cup raw walnuts

1. Place the kale in a large bowl.
2. In a high-powered blender, blend the oranges, cashews, mint, ginger, lemon juice, and dates until smooth and creamy.

3. Pour the dressing over the kale and massage well with tongs. Top with the pomegranate seeds and walnuts and serve. Store leftovers in an airtight container in the refrigerator for up to 1 week.

Substitute it: Use diced stone fruit like plums, peaches, or nectarines in place of oranges when in season.

Per serving: Calories: 305; Total Fat: 17g; Saturated Fat: 2g; Cholesterol: 0mg; Sodium: 16mg; Carbohydrates: 38g; Fiber: 7g; Total Sugar: 24g; Added Sugar: 0g; Protein: 8g; Potassium: 640mg; Magnesium: 94mg; Vitamin K: 234mcg

Zucchini No-Tato Salad

30 Minutes or Less, Gluten-Free
Serves 4 / Prep time: 15 minutes, plus 10 minutes to chill

Potato salad with no potatoes? Yes indeed. And it's still tangy and satisfying. Serve this at your next cookout and help all of your friends and family eat just a little bit healthier.

3 medium zucchini, diced

3 celery stalks, diced

¼ red onion, diced

¼ cup sliced black olives

¼ cup chopped fresh parsley

1 avocado, cubed

3 tablespoons yellow mustard

½ teaspoon garlic powder

Juice of 1 lemon

1. In a large bowl, combine the zucchini, celery, onion, olives, and parsley.
2. In a medium bowl, mash together the avocado, mustard, garlic power, and lemon juice. Stir well to combine.
3. Pour the dressing over the salad and toss to coat. Chill for at least 10 minutes before serving. Store leftovers in an airtight container in the refrigerator for up to 3 days.

Flavor boost: For a fun twist, I like to add fresh or dried dill, sliced cherry tomatoes, corn, and raw pistachios or pumpkin seeds.

Per serving: Calories: 117; Total Fat: 7g; Saturated Fat: 1g; Cholesterol: 0mg; Sodium: 373mg; Carbohydrates: 12g; Fiber: 5g; Total Sugar: 5g; Added Sugar: 0g; Protein: 4g; Potassium: 713mg; Magnesium: 49mg; Vitamin K: 84mcg

Watermelon, Mint, and Lime Salad

5 Ingredients or Fewer, 30 Minutes or Less, Extra-Low Sodium, Gluten-Free, One-Pot
Serves 4 / Prep time: 15 minutes

Watermelon, mint, and lime—what combination could possibly be more refreshing? This salad is perfect pre- and post-workout and as a rejuvenating snack or side dish on a hot summer day. It is also the quickest and easiest crowd-pleaser at any cookout or party.

¼ watermelon, cut into 1-inch cubes

Juice of 1 lime

¼ cup finely chopped fresh mint leaves

1. In a large bowl, gently toss together the watermelon, lime juice, and mint.
2. Serve. Store leftovers in an airtight container in the refrigerator for up to 1 week.

Flavor boost: Diced red onion or scallion make a fun addition to this salad. Another option is to serve this salad over unsweetened vanilla plant-based yogurt.

Per serving: Calories: 24; Total Fat: 0g; Saturated Fat: 0g; Cholesterol: 0mg; Sodium: 2mg; Carbohydrates: 6g; Fiber: 0g; Total Sugar: 4g; Added Sugar: 0g; Protein: 1g; Potassium: 100mg; Magnesium: 7mg; Vitamin K: 0.1mcg

Thai-Inspired Pumpkin Tom Kha Soup

30 Minutes or Less, Gluten-Free
Serves 3 / Prep time: 20 minutes / Cook time: 10 minutes

Tom kha soup is one of my favorite authentic Thai dishes. It is filled with healthy vegetables and is traditionally made with a coconut cream base. This version, made creamy with pumpkin puree, is much more heart healthy and colorful.

For the broth

1 (15-ounce) can unsweetened pumpkin puree

1½ cups unsweetened plain soy milk

1½ tablespoons coconut aminos or reduced-sodium tamari

Juice of 1½ limes

2 pitted Medjool dates

1½-inch piece fresh ginger, peeled

½ tablespoon finely chopped jalapeño

1 small garlic clove, peeled

1 to 2 teaspoons grated lemon zest (optional)

For the veggies

2 cups very thinly sliced kale

½ cup diced red bell pepper

½ cup sliced carrot

½ cup daikon radish, grated or cut into half-moons

To make the broth

1. In a high-powered blender, combine the pumpkin puree, soy milk, coconut aminos, lime juice, dates, ginger, jalapeño, garlic, and lemon zest (if using) and blend for about 1 minute, or until liquefied.

To cook the veggies

2. In a large pot, combine the broth, kale, bell pepper, carrot, and daikon. Bring to a boil over high heat, then reduce to medium-high heat and simmer for 2 to 5 minutes, until heated through.

3. Serve warm. Store leftovers in an airtight container in the refrigerator for up to 1 week or in the freezer for up to 1 month.

Make it easier: Instead of using 2 dates to sweeten the soup, which requires a blender, make this a one-pot meal and use 1 to 2 tablespoons of maple syrup or whatever liquid sweetener you prefer.

Flavor boost: To make this a more balanced meal, I like to add 1 cup of no-salt-added chickpeas or a block of diced tempeh or extra-firm tofu. Add whatever additional veggies you like. Burdock root, red cabbage, squash, and even peas are all fantastic additions. Another option is to try a more traditional version using 2 (15-ounce) cans of full-fat coconut milk instead of the soy milk and pumpkin puree.

Per serving: Calories: 190; Total Fat: 3g; Saturated Fat: 0g; Cholesterol: 0mg; Sodium: 416mg; Carbohydrates: 35g; Fiber: 8g; Total Sugar: 20g; Added Sugar: 0g; Protein: 8g; Potassium: 376mg; Magnesium: 33mg; Vitamin K: 57mcg

Easy Pea Soup

5 Ingredients or Fewer, 30 Minutes or Less, Extra-Low Sodium, Gluten-Free
Serves 2 / Prep time: 5 minutes / Cook time: 20 minutes

Don't underestimate this simple indulgent soup. Peas are the most naturally sweet green vegetable, and they provide impressive protein content with all nine essential amino acids. Anyone with a sensitive stomach or who has a hard time tolerating soy or beans will likely be fine with peas.

3 cups Save-the-Scraps Vegetable Stock (page 142) or store-bought low-sodium vegetable broth

3 cups frozen peas, thawed

1. In a medium pot, bring the stock to a boil. Add the peas and reduce the heat to medium. Cook for 15 minutes, or until the peas are cooked through and tender.

2. Transfer to a high-powered blender and blend until smooth and creamy, 1 to 2 minutes.

3. Pour into two soup bowls and enjoy. Store leftovers in an airtight container in the refrigerator for up to 1 week.

Flavor boost: Add toppings of your choice such as nutritional yeast, Spicy Roasted Chickpeas (page 98), fresh mint, garlic, lemon juice, or toasted sliced almonds.

Per serving: Calories: 210; Total Fat: 1g; Saturated Fat: 0g; Cholesterol: 0mg; Sodium: 25mg; Carbohydrates: 39g; Fiber: 12g; Total Sugar: 12g; Added Sugar: 0g; Protein: 12g; Potassium: 264mg; Magnesium: 53mg; Vitamin K: 58mcg

Simple Miso Soup

5 Ingredients or Fewer, 30 Minutes or Less, Gluten-Free, One-Pot
Serves 4 / Prep time: 20 minutes / Cook time: 10 minutes

Miso soup is a traditional Japanese soup. It can be as simple as just broth and scallions or packed with vegetables and tofu. Miso is a fermented soy paste that is full of savory flavor. Got leftover rice and veggies? Make some miso soup! Purchase no-salt-added microwavable brown rice packets in the frozen aisle of your grocery store to make this recipe quickly.

4 cups water

¼ cup sweet white miso

1 cup cooked brown rice

½ cup chopped scallions

7 ounces (½ block) extra-firm tofu, cubed

1. In a large saucepan, heat the water over medium-low heat. Just before the water comes to a simmer, whisk in the miso. To keep the beneficial probiotic bacteria in the fermented miso alive, keep the heat on low to medium-low and keep from actively simmering or boiling. It is still very healthy if brought to a simmer or boiled, but the extra benefits are preserved if kept a little bit cooler.

2. Add the brown rice, scallions, and tofu. Cook for 2 to 5 minutes, until the rice and tofu are warmed through.

3. Serve warm. Store leftovers in an airtight container in the refrigerator for up to 1 week.

Per serving: Calories: 136; Total Fat: 3g; Saturated Fat: 0.5g; Cholesterol: 0mg; Sodium: 438mg; Carbohydrates: 22g; Fiber: 1g; Total Sugar: 7g; Added Sugar: 0g; Protein: 7g; Potassium: 118mg; Magnesium: 36mg; Vitamin K: 15mcg

Mushroom and Bean Chili

Gluten-Free, One-Pot
Serves 4 / Prep time: 20 minutes / Cook time: 25 minutes

This chili was inspired by a version created by Emeril Lagassé for the Food Network. I made it simpler by using frozen corn instead of chopped zucchini, canned diced tomatoes (I like Muir Glen brand) instead of fresh, plus an addition of prewashed baby spinach. This version is oil- and salt-free of course, without compromising flavor.

1½ cups chopped red onion

1 cup chopped red bell pepper

2 tablespoons minced garlic

3 cups frozen corn, thawed

15 ounces cremini mushrooms, chopped

2 tablespoons salt-free chili powder

1 tablespoon ground cumin

½ teaspoon smoked paprika

2 (14.5-ounce) cans no-salt-added fire-roasted diced tomatoes

3 cups no-salt-added canned black beans, drained and rinsed

1 (15-ounce) can no-salt-added tomato sauce

1 cup Save-the-Scraps Vegetable Stock (page 142), store-bought low-sodium vegetable broth, or water

8 ounces baby spinach

⅓ avocado, sliced, for garnish

1. In a large pot, combine the onions, peppers, and garlic and water-sauté (see page 18) over medium heat, stirring for about 3 minutes, or until soft.

2. Add the corn and mushrooms and cook, stirring, for 5 minutes, or until soft.

3. Stir in the chili powder, cumin, and smoked paprika. Then add the tomatoes with their juices, beans, tomato sauce, and stock. Stir well, increase the heat, and bring to a boil. Reduce the heat to medium-low and simmer, stirring occasionally, for 15 minutes, or until

fragrant and the desired thickness is achieved. The longer the cooking time, the more water will evaporate, providing a thicker stew.

4. Remove from the heat and stir in the spinach. Garnish with avocado and serve. Store leftovers in an airtight container in the refrigerator for up to 1 week or in the freezer for up to 1 month.

Flavor boost: Try adding ½ teaspoon cayenne pepper for an extra kick or in place of the smoked paprika.

Per serving: Calories: 486; Total Fat: 7g; Saturated Fat: 1g; Cholesterol: 0mg; Sodium: 209mg; Carbohydrates: 89g; Fiber: 26g; Total Sugar: 20g; Added Sugar: 0g; Protein: 25g; Potassium: 2,471mg; Magnesium: 232mg; Vitamin K: 293mcg

Butternut Squash Soup

5 Ingredients or Fewer, 30 Minutes or Less, Extra-Low Sodium, Gluten-Free, One-Pot
Serves 2 / Prep time: 5 minutes / Cook time: 25 minutes

What does Thanksgiving taste like? The answer is this soup. Ginger is a potent anti-inflammatory that does wonders for indigestion and migraines. Purchase already peeled and chopped squash to make this recipe come together in just 30 minutes.

3 cups 1-inch cubes butternut squash

2 cup unsweetened plain plant-based milk

½ teaspoon ground cinnamon

½-inch piece fresh ginger, finely minced

1 teaspoon pumpkin pie spice

1. In a large pot, combine the squash, milk, cinnamon, ginger, and pumpkin pie spice and bring to a simmer over medium-high heat. Cook, stirring occasionally, for about 20 minutes, or until the squash is tender.

2. Use an immersion blender (or transfer to a regular blender) and blend until smooth and creamy.

3. Serve warm. Store leftovers in an airtight container in the refrigerator for up to 1 week.

Make it easier: Cook the squash the night before by steaming, boiling, or roasting it. To steam or boil, place chopped squash in a steamer basket above boiling water to steam, or boil directly in the water, for about 30 minutes, or until fork-tender. To roast the squash, preheat the oven to 425°F. Spread the 1-inch chunks over a sheet pan lined with parchment paper. Invert another sheet pan over it to trap the moisture. Bake for 15 minutes. Remove the top pan and bake for another 15 minutes, or until fork-tender.

Per serving: Calories: 203; Total Fat: 4g; Saturated Fat: 1g; Cholesterol: 0mg; Sodium: 87mg; Carbohydrates: 35g; Fiber: 12g; Total Sugar: 7g; Added Sugar: 0g; Protein: 10g; Potassium: 1,223mg; Magnesium: 129mg; Vitamin K: 3mcg

Simple Avocado and Hummus Wraps

30 Minutes or Less, One-Pot
Serves 2 / Prep time: 10 minutes / Cook time: 10 minutes

These rainbow-hued wraps are made with red tomato, orange carrot, and green avocado. If you make them ahead of time, wrap them in parchment paper or put them in an air-tight container.

2 (9-inch) whole-grain tortillas, homemade (page 106) or store-bought

⅓ cup Spicy Roasted Red Pepper Hummus (page 100) or store-bought hummus

½ avocado, sliced

2 cup mixed baby greens or chopped lettuce

1 small or medium tomato, sliced

½ cup shredded carrots

1. In a medium skillet, heat the tortillas over medium heat for 1 to 2 minutes on each side, until they reach your desired crispness.

2. Spread the hummus, avocado, greens, tomato, and carrots evenly over both tortillas.

3. Roll up, cut in half, and serve immediately.

Substitute it: Instead of flour tortillas, make wraps with collard leaves: Trim the stems off of 2 collard leaves just where the stem goes past the leaves. Horizontally slice off the top of the midrib to make the leaf more pliable.

Per serving (1 wrap): Calories: 267; Total Fat: 11g; Saturated Fat: 1g; Cholesterol: 0mg; Sodium: 160mg; Carbohydrates: 28g; Fiber: 10g; Total Sugar: 5g; Added Sugar: 0g; Protein: 8g; Potassium: 693mg; Magnesium: 202mg; Vitamin K: 65mcg

Three-Ingredient No-Queso-Dillas

5 Ingredients or Fewer, 30 Minutes or Less
Serves 3 / Prep time: 5 minutes / Cook time: 25 minutes

Pile that spinach *high* and watch a mountain of spinach disappear within minutes. Trust me, it will cook down to an amount that looks realistic to eat. These are so fun and easy to make, and you'll get iron, fiber, and protein in a mineral-packed punch from the greens and beans. I like Ezekiel 4:9 brand tortillas. To lower the sodium in this recipe, skip the store-bought salsa and instead top your quesadillas with a scoop of Tomato and Corn Fiesta Salad (page 44).

8 cups spinach (or greens of choice)

2 (15-ounce) cans no-salt-added pinto beans (or bean of choice), drained and rinsed

6 whole-grain tortillas, homemade (page 106) or store-bought

Avocado oil cooking spray

1 cup salsa

1. In a large skillet, water-sauté (see page 18) the spinach over medium heat for about 5 minutes, or until wilted, adding water as needed to prevent burning.

2. In a medium bowl, mash the beans with a potato masher or fork. Add the spinach and mix until well combined.

3. Spread one-third of the bean/spinach mixture on a tortilla and place another tortilla on top. Repeat until you've made 3 quesadillas.

4. Mist a medium skillet with oil and set over medium heat. Warm each quesadilla for 2 to 3 minutes on each side, until golden brown and crispy on the edges.

5. Cut each quesadilla into quarters and serve with ⅓ cup salsa.

Substitute it: Add your favorite mock meat, tempeh, or tofu, try mashed sweet potato instead of beans, or use sautéed mushrooms or kale instead of spinach.

Per serving: Calories: 520; Total Fat: 4g; Saturated Fat: 0g; Cholesterol: 0mg; Sodium: 432mg; Carbohydrates: 101g; Fiber: 23g; Total Sugar: 1g; Added Sugar: 0g; Protein: 26g; Potassium: 1408mg; Magnesium: 477mg; Vitamin K: 392mcg

BBQ Tempeh Wraps

30 Minutes or Less, Gluten-Free

Serves 2 / Prep time: 10 minutes / Cook time: 20 minutes

Tempah is made with soybeans, so it is slightly less processed and has a meatier texture than tofu. I like Primal Kitchen brand barbecue sauce if I don't have any homemade on hand, but you can try this with any sauce you like. To reduce the sodium content, use less barbecue sauce.

1 (8-ounce) package tempeh, sliced into thin strips

1 cup BBQ Sauce (page 138) or store-bought low-sodium barbecue sauce

½ cup plain plant-based yogurt, store-bought or homemade (page 144), or Tzatziki (page 137)

2 (9-inch) whole-grain tortillas, homemade (page 106) or store-bought

½ cucumber, thinly sliced

½ carrot, grated

½ avocado, sliced

1. Preheat the oven to 350°F. Line a rimmed baking sheet with parchment paper.

2. In a medium bowl, combine the tempeh and barbecue sauce and toss until well coated.

3. Evenly distribute the tempeh on the baking sheet and bake for 15 to 20 minutes, until the tempeh has absorbed the sauce.

4. To assemble, spread ¼ cup yogurt or tzatziki over each tortilla. Then, dividing evenly, top the tortillas with tempeh, sliced cucumbers, grated carrot, and avocado. Fold in the sides and roll up tightly.

5. Cut in half and serve immediately. Or, if desired, heat the wraps in a medium skillet over medium heat for 2 minutes on each side, or until warmed through, then cut in half.

Make it easier: Don't want to wait 15 to 20 minutes for the tempeh to bake? In a medium to large saucepan, combine the barbecue sauce and sliced tempeh and stir over medium heat for about 5 minutes, or until the tempeh soaks up the sauce.

Per serving (1 wrap): Calories: 619; Total Fat: 16g; Saturated Fat: 2g; Cholesterol: 0mg; Sodium: 302mg; Carbohydrates: 84g; Fiber: 10g; Total Sugar: 33g; Added Sugar: 0g; Protein: 31g; Potassium: 1407mg; Magnesium: 331mg; Vitamin K: 21mcg

Cauliflower "Tuna"

30 Minutes or Less, Gluten-Free
Serves 3 / Prep time: 10 minutes / Cook time: 10 minutes

My friends tell me they like this better than actual tuna, which is fantastic because overfishing of the oceans is at an all-time high. This alternative provides a lot more fiber, flavor, and texture than traditional tuna and will certainly satisfy. I first saw a version of this recipe on *Forks Over Knives*, but this version is made with cauliflower instead of chickpeas and has a significant source of iodine from the dulse or kelp granules, which also provide an added fishy taste. For the mustard, look for one that is less than 140mg sodium per serving.

1 small head cauliflower, broken into florets

2 teaspoons no-salt-added spicy brown or Dijon mustard

3 tablespoons tahini

Juice of ½ lemon

¼ teaspoon red pepper flakes

¼ teaspoon freshly ground black pepper

⅓ cup diced onion

⅓ cup diced dill pickle

⅓ cup diced celery

¼ cup chopped fresh parsley

1 teaspoon sea vegetable (dulse or kelp) granules

1. In a pot fitted with a steamer basket, bring water to a boil and steam the cauliflower for 7 minutes, or until fork-tender but not mushy.

2. Measure out 2 cups steamed cauliflower and transfer to a large bowl (2 cups steamed cauliflower reduces to about 1½ cups mashed). Mash the cauliflower with a fork, leaving some larger pieces as desired for texture.

3. Stir in the mustard, tahini, lemon juice, pepper flakes, black pepper, onion, pickle, celery, parsley, and sea vegetable granules.

4. Enjoy. Store leftovers in an airtight container in the refrigerator for up to 1 week.

Flavor boost: Serve over greens or use it as filling in a sandwich. Try adding sliced grapes, diced tomatoes, and roasted sunflower seeds for an extra pop of flavor and texture. This "tuna" is also fantastic with other fresh herbs like cilantro, dill, or basil, along with Beet Spread (page 139) or Lemon-Tahini Dressing (page 141). It goes well on toasted bread, in a pita, or in a tortilla (page 106) along with lettuce, tomato, onion, avocado, and more mustard and pickle.

Substitute it: Instead of the cauliflower, mash 1 (15-ounce) can of no-salt-added drained and rinsed white beans, pinto beans, chickpeas, or lentils (or 1½ cups of home-cooked beans).

Per serving: Calories: 125; Total Fat: 9g; Saturated Fat: 1g; Cholesterol: 0mg; Sodium: 260mg; Carbohydrates: 10g; Fiber: 4g; Total Sugar: 3g; Added Sugar: 0g; Protein: 5g; Potassium: 288mg; Magnesium: 30mg; Vitamin K: 99mcg

Seven-Layer Dip Burrito

30 Minutes or Less, One-Pot
Serves 4 / Prep time: 15 minutes

I could not have made it through college without Chipotle. If you want an even fresher and quicker version of their burritos that's lower in sodium and just as tasty with even more veggies, this is the recipe for you. I like Ezekiel 4:9 brand tortillas and Amy's "light in sodium" vegetarian refried beans.

4 (9-inch) whole-grain tortillas, homemade (page 106) or store-bought

4 cups shredded romaine lettuce

1 cup low-fat, low-sodium refried beans

4 tablespoons chopped olives

2 tablespoons minced jalapeño

½ cup salsa

½ cup corn kernels, fresh or thawed frozen

1 avocado, sliced

½ cup shredded carrots

4 tablespoons plain soy yogurt (optional)

1. Dividing evenly, fill the tortillas with romaine, refried beans, olives, jalapeño, salsa, corn, avocado, and carrots.

2. Top each with 1 tablespoon yogurt (if using). Roll up and enjoy immediately.

Substitute it: Don't have refried beans? Drain the liquid from a can of chickpeas (this is called aquafaba) and set it aside. Mash or blend 1¼ to 1½ cups of beans. In a medium skillet. sauté the mashed beans in ¼ cup of aquafaba over medium-high heat, along with ¼ cup of diced onion and 2 minced garlic cloves or ½ teaspoon of garlic powder. Cook for 5 to 10 minutes, until the onions are translucent. If you prefer, you can use vegetable broth instead of the aquafaba.

Per serving: Calories: 282; Total Fat: 12g; Saturated Fat: 2g; Cholesterol: 0mg; Sodium: 215mg; Carbohydrates: 44g; Fiber: 11g; Total Sugar: 2g; Added Sugar: 0g; Protein: 10g; Potassium: 747mg; Magnesium: 232mg; Vitamin K: 60mcg

TLT and Avocado Panini

30 Minutes or Less, One-Pot
Serves 4 / Prep time: 15 minutes / Cook time: 10 minutes

Love BLT sandwiches? Well, I hate to burst your bacon bubble, but according to a recent study, bacon, among other processed foods, can increase your risk of death from heart disease by 58 percent. No amount of greasy deliciousness is worth that statistic.

¼ cup Save-the-Scraps Vegetable Stock (page 142) or store-bought low-sodium vegetable broth

½ teaspoon dried oregano

½ teaspoon paprika

¼ teaspoon garlic powder

¼ teaspoon onion powder

2 (8-ounce) packages tempeh, sliced

8 slices whole-grain sourdough bread

1 avocado, sliced

1 tomato

Sliced lettuce

1. In a medium skillet, combine the broth, oregano, paprika, garlic powder, and onion powder and mix well. Set the skillet over medium heat, add the tempeh, and sauté for 2 to 5 minutes, until the tempeh has soaked up the liquid and is tender.

2. Toast the bread (if desired) and spread one-quarter of the avocado on each of 4 slices of bread. Layer the tempeh slices and tomato and lettuce and top each sandwich with the other 4 slices of bread. Enjoy immediately.

Flavor boost: To make this sandwich extra special, add fresh basil and sautéed spinach. To make the tempeh taste more like bacon, add a little coconut aminos or reduced-sodium tamari, liquid smoke, and black pepper.

Per serving: Calories: 453; Total Fat: 19g; Saturated Fat: 4g; Cholesterol: 0mg; Sodium: 397mg; Carbohydrates: 46g; Fiber: 9g; Total Sugar: 7g; Added Sugar: 0g; Protein: 31g; Potassium: 801mg; Magnesium: 126mg; Vitamin K: 33mcg

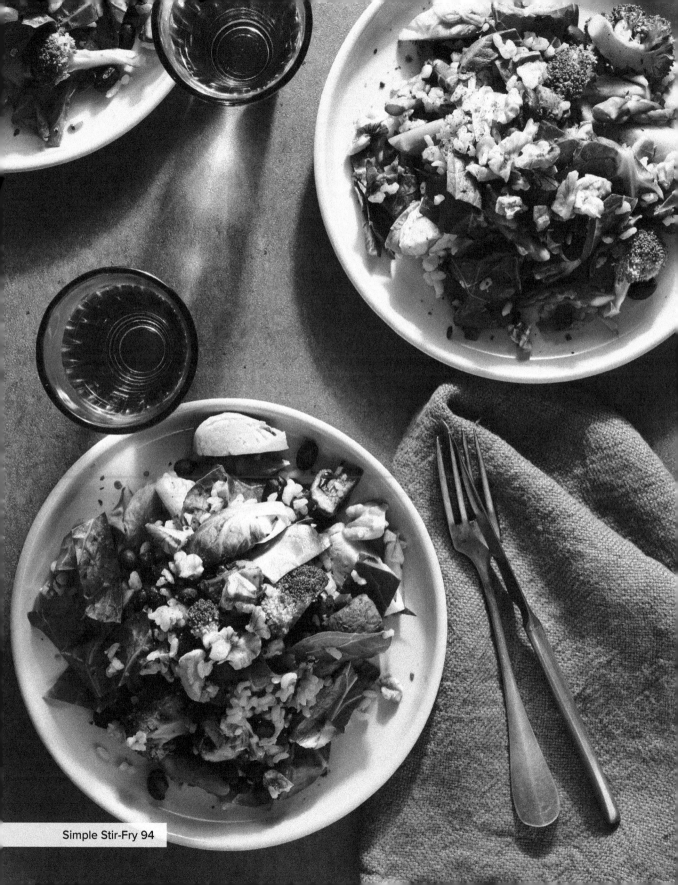

4

Main Meals

Red Curry

30 Minutes or Less, Gluten-Free
Serves 8 / Prep time: 10 minutes / Cook time: 20 minutes

When I first moved to California, I cooked for retreats all over Los Angeles and Hawaii. Everyone's favorite dinner? This curry. It's an all-around favorite because it is time-efficient and uses up leftover vegetables, and even people with varying food preferences love it! If possible, soak the rice before rinsing and cooking: Combine 2 cups of rice with 4 cups of filtered water and soak overnight in the refrigerator to save time when making the dish. I like Thai Kitchen brand red curry paste.

4 cups water

2 cups brown rice, soaked overnight and drained

2 (13.5-ounce) cans full-fat coconut milk

½ cup Thai red curry paste

1 small onion, chopped

3 garlic cloves, minced

1 tablespoon minced fresh ginger

1½ cups chopped broccoli florets

1 pound mushrooms, chopped

1½ pounds tempeh or tofu, cut into cubes

1. In a medium saucepan, bring the water to a boil. Add the rice, reduce the heat to a simmer, and cook until the water is absorbed, about 20 minutes, stirring occasionally.

2. Meanwhile, in a large pot, whisk together the coconut milk and curry paste. Add the onion, garlic, and ginger and simmer over medium heat for 2 to 5 minutes, until fragrant and the onion is translucent.

3. Add the broccoli, mushrooms, and tempeh or tofu and let simmer for another 5 to 10 minutes, until all the vegetables are cooked.

4. Serve the curry with a side of cooked brown rice. Store leftovers in an airtight container in the refrigerator for up to 1 week or in the freezer for up to 2 months.

Substitute it: Reduce the fat content by replacing 1 can of coconut milk with 1 can of pumpkin puree. Also, use whatever vegetables you have in the fridge, and if you prefer Thai green or yellow curry pastes, try those. When I use tofu for this recipe, I prefer it to be quite firm. I like my tofu pressed—I think it improves the texture. You can find tofu presses online for about $30.

Per serving: Calories: 529; Total Fat: 24g; Saturated Fat: 16g; Cholesterol: 0mg; Sodium: 417mg; Carbohydrates: 51g; Fiber: 11g; Total Sugar: 6g; Added Sugar: 0g; Protein: 23g; Potassium: 650mg; Magnesium: 52mg; Vitamin K: 17mcg

Crispy Baked Tofu Pad Thai

5 Ingredients or Fewer, Extra-Low Sodium, Gluten-Free
Serves 4 / Prep time: 10 minutes / Cook time: 40 minutes

This meal is great if you already have Peanut Sauce (page 140) in the refrigerator. I didn't like tofu until I tried it baked like this. If you think you don't like tofu, keep trying different cooking methods and sauces.

8 ounces pad Thai rice noodles

1 (14-ounce) block extra-firm tofu

1 cup Peanut Sauce (page 140)

1 red bell pepper, thinly sliced

¼ cup water

6 cups chopped kale (or other pre-ferred green)

4 tablespoons unsalted roasted peanuts, chopped (optional)

1. Preheat the oven to 425°F. Line a rimmed baking sheet with parchment paper or a silicone baking mat.

2. Meanwhile, cook the rice noodles according to the package directions and set aside.

3. Drain the tofu, wrap in a kitchen towel, and gently but firmly squeeze it to remove as much liquid as possible; take care not to break the tofu apart. Cut the tofu into small cubes. (The smaller the cubes, the less cooking time.) Distribute the tofu evenly over the baking sheet and bake for 15 minutes; flip and bake for 10 to 15 minutes more.

4. In a large skillet or wok, combine the peanut sauce, rice noodles, baked tofu, and bell pepper. Mix over medium heat for about 2 minutes, or until well combined.

5. In a medium skillet, heat the water over medium-high and add the chopped greens to steam them, stirring frequently, for about 5 minutes, or until wilted.

6. Serve the pad Thai over the steamed greens, garnishing each serving with 1 tablespoon roasted peanuts (if using). Store leftovers in an airtight container in the refrigerator for up to 1 week.

Flavor boost: Before combining the noodles, tofu, and Peanut Sauce, water-sauté (see page 18) 2 medium carrots (thinly sliced), 1 cup of roughly chopped broccoli, and the bell pepper for about 5 minutes. Then garnish with fresh scallions and a squeeze of lime juice.

Make it easier: Have an air fryer? You can make crispy tofu in about 10 minutes. And to make firmer tofu, instead of squeezing by hand, purchase a tofu press online. Pressed tofu makes a world of difference with texture. Another way to press tofu is to leave it in the refrigerator, wrapped in clean towels with something heavy on top, like a glass baking dish. Simple, but it does the trick! If you prefer, steam the greens in a steamer pot or covered in the microwave in a microwave-safe bowl with some water.

Per serving: Calories: 512; Total Fat: 19g; Saturated Fat: 3g; Cholesterol: 0mg; Sodium: 112mg; Carbohydrates: 69g; Fiber: 5g; Total Sugar: 16g; Added Sugar: 0g; Protein: 22g; Potassium: 529mg; Magnesium: 106mg; Vitamin K: 5mcg

Five-Ingredient Beet Burgers

5 Ingredients or Fewer, Extra-Low Sodium, Gluten-Free
Makes 8 burgers / Prep time: 20 minutes / Cook time: 50 minutes

Beets are included in many of my recipes because they are an incredible source of nitrates, which have been shown to significantly improve cardiovascular health and oxygen utilization. These burgers require a bit of work, so double the recipe and freeze extra patties to enjoy anytime. If you don't already have cooked quinoa on-hand, you can use store-bought frozen quinoa in a pinch.

2 to 2⅔ cups grated beets (1 large or 2 small beets)

1 large onion, diced

2 to 2½ teaspoons smoked paprika

1⅓ cups pumpkin seeds

2 cups cooked quinoa

1. Preheat the oven to 350°F. Line a rimmed baking sheet with parchment paper.

2. Squeeze the excess liquid from the grated beets, place them in a large bowl, and set aside.

3. In a medium skillet, water-sauté (see page 18) the onion over medium-high heat for 2 to 5 minutes, adding more water as needed. Once the onions are soft and translucent, stir in the smoked paprika and mix for another minute. Remove from the heat and set aside.

4. In a food processor, combine the pumpkin seeds and cooked quinoa and process until thick and smooth. Add half the beets and the sautéed onion and pulse until just combined.

5. Transfer the mixture to the bowl with the rest of the grated beets and mix until well combined. The mixture should be firm, slightly sticky, and easily formed into patties.

6. Divide and form the mixture into 8 patties. Place the patties on the baking sheet and bake for about 45 minutes, or until golden and crispy on top.

7. Serve warm. Store leftovers in an airtight container in the refrigerator for up to 1 week or in the freezer for up to 2 months.

Flavor boost: Add salt-free chili powder, cayenne pepper, or coconut aminos for an extra kick. Serve these patties with BBQ Sauce (page 138) or Tzatziki (page 137), lettuce, and sliced cucumber on toasted whole-wheat buns.

Per serving (1 burger): Calories: 222; Total Fat: 10g; Saturated Fat: 2g; Cholesterol: 0mg; Sodium: 78mg; Carbohydrates: 24g; Fiber: 6g; Total Sugar: 8g; Added Sugar: 0g; Protein: 11g; Potassium: 587mg; Magnesium: 55mg; Vitamin K: 1mcg

Buffalo Cauliflower Macaroni

30 Minutes or Less, Extra-Low Sodium
Serves 4 / Prep time: 10 minutes / Cook time: 20 minutes

Goodbye butter, milk, and cheese. Hello tofu, cashews, and cauliflower! Whoever thinks they are "too old" to say macaroni and cheese is their favorite food clearly never tried this dish. Purchase prechopped cauliflower to make this recipe quick and easy. To pack in plenty of nutrients and make the dish gluten-free, use a bean-based elbow macaroni, such as Banza elbows, which are made from chickpea flour. I like Siete brand hot sauce for this recipe.

4 cups chopped cauliflower florets

8 ounces whole-grain elbow macaroni

1 (14-ounce) block firm tofu, drained

½ cup raw cashews

1 teaspoon smoked paprika

3 tablespoons hot sauce

4 teaspoons apple cider vinegar

2 garlic cloves, peeled

⅛ teaspoon freshly ground black pepper

Pinch cayenne pepper

1. Preheat the oven to 450°F. Line a rimmed baking sheet with parchment paper or a silicone baking mat.

2. Spread the cauliflower on the baking sheet and invert a second baking sheet on top. Bake for 10 minutes. Remove the top baking sheet and bake for 10 more minutes, or until golden and tender.

3. While the cauliflower cooks, cook the pasta according to the package directions. Drain and return to the pot.

4. Meanwhile, in a high-powered blender or food processor, blend the tofu, cashews, smoked paprika, hot sauce, vinegar, garlic, black pepper, and cayenne until smooth, 1 to 2 minutes.

5. To the pot with the cooked noodles, add the cauliflower and sauce and mix well.

6. Serve warm. Store leftovers in an airtight container in the refrigerator for up to 1 week.

Flavor boost: Mix in asparagus or broccoli with the cauliflower, as well as Spicy Roasted Chickpeas (page 98), and top with Three-Seed "Parmesan" (page 135). Or serve the sauce over steamed spinach, kale, or collard greens with extra hot sauce or cayenne and garnish with chopped fresh herbs or scallions.

Per serving: Calories: 403; Total Fat: 14g; Saturated Fat: 3g; Cholesterol: 0mg; Sodium: 120mg; Carbohydrates: 56g; Fiber: 9g; Total Sugar: 4g; Added Sugar: 0g; Protein: 22g; Potassium: 749mg; Magnesium: 1892mg; Vitamin K: 26mcg

Red Rice, Mango, and Black Bean Bowl

30 Minutes or Less, Extra-Low Sodium, Gluten-Free, One-Pot
Serves 4 / Prep time: 15 minutes / Cook time: 5 minutes

Combining spicy with sweet is a great way to boost flavor without adding salt. I also recommend garnishing with a healthy source of fat—such as the avocado in this dish—to soothe the heat from the spice. If you don't have leftover cooked brown rice, use microwavable frozen brown rice.

2 cups cooked brown rice

½ cup no-salt-added tomato sauce

½ teaspoon salt-free chili powder

4 cups chopped romaine lettuce

2 (15-ounce) cans no-salt-added black beans, drained and rinsed

1⅓ cups frozen mango chunks, thawed and diced (or 2 mangos, diced)

1 red bell pepper, diced

1 avocado, sliced

1 cup chopped fresh cilantro

2 limes, halved, for serving

1. In a medium skillet, combine the rice, tomato sauce, and chili powder and mix well. Cook over medium-high heat for 2 to 5 minutes, until fragrant and well combined. Remove from the heat.

2. Dividing evenly, make layers in four bowls in this order: lettuce, red rice mixture, black beans, mango, bell pepper, avocado slices, and cilantro.

3. Serve with lime halves for squeezing. Store leftovers in an airtight container in the refrigerator for up to 1 week.

Flavor boost: Add ½ cup of Tomato and Corn Fiesta Salad (page 44).

Substitute it: Fresh or frozen (thawed) pineapple also works well instead of mango in this recipe. If you don't have cooked rice or store-bought frozen rice, bring 2 cups of low-sodium vegetable broth to a boil over high heat. Add 1 cup of brown rice, reduce to a simmer, cover, and cook, stirring occasionally, until the rice is tender and the water is absorbed, about 45 minutes.

Per serving: Calories: 441; Total Fat: 7g; Saturated Fat: 1g; Cholesterol: 0mg; Sodium: 33mg; Carbohydrates: 82g; Fiber: 21g; Total Sugar: 15g; Added Sugar: 0g; Protein: 16g; Potassium: 1,066mg; Magnesium: 131mg; Vitamin K: 72mcg

Creamy Sweet Potato and Pea Curry

30 Minutes or Less, Gluten-Free, One-Pot
Serves 4 / Prep time: 15 minutes / Cook time: 15 minutes

Nothing is more comforting than a bowl of this curry. Serve it with Homemade Flour Tortillas (page 106) or a side of rice.

1½ cups unsweetened plain soy milk

2 medium sweet potatoes, diced (about 2 cups)

1 large carrot, chopped (about ½ cup)

1 teaspoon red pepper flakes

2 teaspoons curry powder

¼ cup chopped scallions

3 tablespoons unsalted, unsweetened almond butter

¼ cup chopped raw pecans or almonds or unsalted roasted hazelnuts

1½ cups frozen peas, thawed

1 teaspoon coconut aminos, reduced-sodium tamari, or gluten-free soy sauce

1. In a large pot, combine the soy milk, sweet potatoes, and carrot and simmer over medium heat, stirring frequently, for 5 to 10 minutes, until fork-tender.

2. Stir in the pepper flakes, curry powder, scallions, almond butter, chopped nuts, peas, and coconut aminos. Continue stirring, bring to a boil, then remove from the heat.

3. Serve warm. Store leftovers in an airtight container in the refrigerator for up to 1 week.

Substitute it: To add more protein, substitute 1 cup Spicy Roasted Chickpeas (page 98), cubed tempeh, or extra-firm tofu for 1 cup of the sweet potatoes.

Per serving: Calories: 324; Total Fat: 13g; Saturated Fat: 1g; Cholesterol: 0mg; Sodium: 217mg; Carbohydrates: 42g; Fiber: 11g; Total Sugar: 11g; Added Sugar: 0g; Protein: 11g; Potassium: 844mg; Magnesium: 109mg; Vitamin K: 27mcg

Orange Seitan

5 Ingredients or Fewer, 30 Minutes or Less
Serves 3 / Prep time: 10 minutes / Cook time: 5 minutes

Seitan is made from a wheat protein called vital wheat gluten, mixed with water. It has a chewy, meaty texture and flavor. Give it a try! If you are gluten sensitive or intolerant or simply are not a fan of seitan's unique texture, substitute tempeh or baked tofu cubes. It is also fun to make orange cauliflower using baked cauliflower florets in this sauce instead of seitan.

1 cup orange juice

1 tablespoon minced fresh ginger

2 tablespoons coconut aminos or reduced-sodium soy sauce or tamari

1 tablespoon maple syrup

8 ounces traditional seitan

1. In a large bowl, combine the orange juice, ginger, coconut aminos, and maple syrup. Add the seitan and coat well.

2. In a large skillet, stir-fry the seitan and orange sauce over medium-high heat for about 5 minutes, or until the liquid is thickened.

3. Serve warm. Store leftovers in an airtight container in the refrigerator for up to 1 week.

Flavor boost: Add 2 minced garlic cloves, 1 to 2 teaspoons of apple cider vinegar, ½ teaspoon of ground coriander, and freshly ground black pepper to taste.

Per serving: Calories: 146; Total Fat: 1g; Saturated Fat: 0g; Cholesterol: 0mg; Sodium: 195mg; Carbohydrates: 18g; Fiber: 0g; Total Sugar: 11g; Added Sugar: 4g; Protein: 18g; Potassium: 245mg; Magnesium: 21mg; Vitamin K: 0mcg

Bright Baked Falafel

Gluten-Free
Serves 6 / Prep time: 25 minutes / Cook time: 20 minutes

I've been to Israel twice and I still dream about the fresh deep-fried falafel I had there. This baked version provides a rejuvenating freshness with the orange, parsley, lemon, and garlic and lifts you up instead of weighing you down. Enjoy these falafel with friends or have plenty stacked in the refrigerator for a quick fix of filling flavor.

⅔ cup raw pumpkin seeds

5 or 6 pitted Medjool dates

½ orange, peeled

1 cup fresh parsley or cilantro

8 garlic cloves, peeled

Juice of 1 lemon

1½ tablespoons ground cumin

2 (15-ounce) cans no-salt-added chickpeas, drained, rinsed, and patted dry

¼ to ½ cup chickpea flour

1. Preheat the oven to 375°F. Line a rimmed baking sheet with parchment paper or a silicone baking mat.

2. In a food processor, combine the pumpkin seeds, dates, orange, parsley, garlic, lemon juice, and cumin and pulse until just until roughly chopped. Stop once or twice to scrape down the sides with a rubber spatula.

3. Add the chickpeas to the food processor. Blend the ingredients, scrape down the sides with a rubber spatula, and blend again a few times until the chickpeas are well incorporated.

4. Blend in chickpea flour, 1 tablespoon at a time, starting with the smaller amount. The falafel dough should not stick to your hands. Blend in more flour if the dough is too sticky.

5. Divide and roll the mixture into 24 balls (about a heaping tablespoon each). Arrange on the lined baking sheet and bake for 15 to 20 minutes, until golden and cracked and the falafel easily and cleanly release from the pan.

6. Serve warm. Store leftovers in an airtight container in the refrigerator for up to 1 week.

Flavor boost: Add ½ tablespoon ground turmeric and ⅛ teaspoon freshly ground black pepper for extra health benefits and a beautiful bright yellow color. Serve inside pita bread or Homemade Flour Tortillas (page 106) with chopped romaine lettuce, tomato, cucumber, Tzatziki (page 137), Beet Spread (page 139), Spicy Roasted Red Pepper Hummus (page 100), or Lemon-Tahini Dressing (page 141).

Per serving: Calories: 282; Total Fat: 9g; Saturated Fat: 1g; Cholesterol: 0mg; Sodium: 173mg; Carbohydrates: 43g; Fiber: 9g; Total Sugar: 19g; Added Sugar: 0g; Protein: 12g; Potassium: 524mg; Magnesium: 117mg; Vitamin K: 168mcg

Squash and Chickpea Harvest Bowl

30 Minutes or Less, Gluten-Free
Serves 4 / Prep time: 10 minutes / Cook time: 20 minutes

My first vegan restaurant experience was at the Organic Garden Cafe in Beverly, Massachusetts, where I had the Harvest Bowl. This much simpler version of that divine meal is just as satisfying.

For the quinoa and squash

3 cups water

1 cup quinoa

2 cups diced peeled butternut squash

For the dressing

Juice of 1 lemon

½ cup orange juice

¼ cup plus 2 tablespoons unsalted, unsweetened almond butter

4 teaspoons curry powder

2 teaspoons red pepper flakes

For the bowls

8 cups packed baby spinach

2 cups no-salt-added canned chickpeas, drained and rinsed, or Spicy Roasted Chickpeas (page 98)

½ cup raw walnuts or pumpkin seeds

½ cup raisins or pomegranate seeds (optional)

To cook the quinoa and squash

1. In a medium saucepan, bring the water to a boil. Add the quinoa, reduce to a simmer, and cook for 15 minutes, or until the water is absorbed and the quinoa is light and fluffy. Remove from the heat and cover to keep warm.

2. Meanwhile, in a large saucepan, water-sauté (see page 18) the squash over medium-high heat for about 10 minutes, or until soft and fork-tender, adding water as needed to prevent burning.

To make the dressing

3. In a medium bowl, whisk together the lemon juice, orange juice, almond butter, curry powder, and pepper flakes.

To assemble the bowls

4. Dividing evenly, in each of four bowls, layer in this order: baby spinach, cooked quinoa, squash, chickpeas, walnuts, and raisins (if using). Drizzle with dressing.

5. Enjoy. Store leftovers in an airtight container in the refrigerator for up to 1 week.

Flavor boost: Make a warm version by stir-frying the squash, quinoa, chickpeas, and spinach in a pan. Then separate the mixture into four bowls and top each with 2 tablespoons of walnuts.

Per serving: Calories: 534; Total Fat: 27g; Saturated Fat: 2g; Cholesterol: 0mg; Sodium: 223mg; Carbohydrates: 61g; Fiber: 17g; Total Sugar: 11g; Added Sugar: 0g; Protein: 20g; Potassium: 1,207mg; Magnesium: 254mg; Vitamin K: 296mcg

Lemon and Herb Tofu Fillets

30 Minutes or Less, Extra-Low Sodium, Gluten-Free
Serves 4 / Prep time: 10 minutes / Cook time: 10 minutes

It's not fish or beef, but it's definitely a delicious fillet. Tofu is quite versatile: It can be crispy, crunchy, or silky smooth, and it can pack a punch of flavor, or not, depending how you prepare it. Keep experimenting with this recipe until the tofu fillet's texture and taste are to your liking. Serve this as you would tilapia or salmon, and add a side of Maple-Balsamic Roasted Veggies (page 108), Quinoa-Pomegranate Holiday Salad (page 45), and Tzatziki (page 137).

1 (14-ounce) block extra-firm tofu

1 teaspoon ground sage

½ teaspoon garlic powder

½ teaspoon dried thyme

½ teaspoon freshly ground black pepper

3 tablespoons balsamic vinegar

Juice of 1 lemon

1. Drain the tofu. Wrap it in a kitchen towel and gently but firmly press the tofu to firm it up; take care not to break the tofu up. Dry it with a clean towel and cut the block of tofu horizontally into 4 slabs ("fillets").

2. In a small bowl, mix together the sage, garlic powder, thyme, pepper, vinegar, and lemon juice. One at a time, coat the tofu fillets in this mixture.

3. In a skillet, cook the fillets over medium heat for 2 minutes on each side, or until the marinade is soaked up. Drizzle any extra marinade over the fillets as they cook. (Alternatively, you can place them on a parchment-lined baking sheet, drizzle with any extra marinade, and bake in a 350°F oven for 10 minutes on each side, or until they reach the desired texture and the marinade is absorbed. Drizzle any extra marinade on top before cooking.)

4. Serve warm. Store leftovers in an airtight container in the refrigerator for up to 1 week.

Flavor boost: For extra *extra* firm fillets, wrap the drained tofu block in a towel and place it in the fridge overnight with something heavy on it, like a glass baking dish. This drastically changes the texture.

Per serving: Calories: 110; Total Fat: 6g; Saturated Fat: 1g; Cholesterol: 0mg; Sodium: 8mg; Carbohydrates: 5g; Fiber: 1g; Total Sugar: 3g; Added Sugar: 0g; Protein: 12g; Potassium: 184mg; Magnesium: 43mg; Vitamin K: 7mcg

Tempeh and Pineapple "Chorizo"

30 Minutes or Less, Gluten-Free, One-Pot
Serves 4 / Prep time: 20 minutes / Cook time: 10 minutes

If you thought salt-free vegan food didn't have any flavor, this spicy tempeh mixed with sweet pineapple will change your mind. Invite some friends over for Taco Tuesday and watch their eyes widen with disbelief. Warm 8 corn tortillas in the microwave or on the stovetop, and serve each taco with ¼ cup of shredded lettuce, 2 tablespoons of diced tomato, ¼ cup of "chorizo," ⅛ avocado, and the juice of ¼ lime. Top with salsa or hot sauce if desired. Or, serve wrapped in red cabbage, lettuce, or collard leaves, over a salad, or simply with rice.

Juice of 1 lemon	1 small red onion, diced
1½ tablespoons sweet white miso paste	5 cremini mushrooms, roughly chopped
½ cup water	2 celery stalks, diced
3 tablespoons salt-free taco seasoning or chili powder	1 (14-ounce) block tempeh, broken into pieces
2 tablespoons nutritional yeast	½ cup frozen pineapple chunks, thawed and chopped into small pieces
3 garlic cloves, minced	⅓ cup chopped walnuts
¼ teaspoon cayenne pepper	

1. In a medium saucepan. stir together the lemon juice, miso, and water. Stir in the taco seasoning, nutritional yeast, garlic, and cayenne.

2. Heat the mixture over medium-high heat, then add the onion, mushrooms, celery, tempeh, and pineapple. Sauté, stirring frequently and adding water, 2 tablespoons at a time, as needed to prevent burning, for 5 to 10 minutes, until the vegetables are cooked through.

3. Remove from the heat and stir in the walnuts.

4. Serve warm. Store leftovers in an airtight container in the refrigerator for up to 1 week.

Substitute it: No tempeh? Try mashed no-salt-added black beans, pinto beans, chickpeas, or Spicy Roasted Chickpeas (page 98). The texture of well-drained extra-firm tofu also works well in this recipe.

Per serving: Calories: 242; Total Fat: 13g; Saturated Fat: 2g; Cholesterol: 0mg; Sodium: 232mg; Carbohydrates: 20g; Fiber: 6g; Total Sugar: 7g; Added Sugar: 0g; Protein: 18g; Potassium: 544mg; Magnesium: 69mg; Vitamin K: 17mcg

Hawaiian Pizzas

30 Minutes or Less, Gluten-Free
Serves 4 / Prep time: 15 minutes / Cook time: 15 minutes

I was initially nervous about going vegan, mostly because: pizza. But since transitioning to a plant-based lifestyle, vegan pizza is one of the meals I make most frequently. For cheese, I like Violife vegan Parmesan or Miyoko's Creamery vegan mozzarella. And for a store-bought BBQ sauce, I like Primal Kitchen unsweetened barbecue sauce.

½ cup BBQ Sauce (page 138) or store-bought low-sodium barbecue sauce

2 frozen store-bought pizza crusts (I like Banza's chickpea crusts)

1 cup thinly sliced red onion

1 cup diced red bell pepper

⅔ cup frozen pineapple chunks, thawed and chopped

1 jalapeño, chopped

¼ cup Herbed Chickpea Spread (page 136) or store-bought vegan cheese

10 slices Tofurky hickory-smoked plant-based deli slices, chopped into bits (optional)

1. Preheat the oven to 350°F. Line two rimmed baking sheets with parchment paper.

2. Spread ¼ cup BBQ sauce evenly over each pizza crust. Dividing evenly, sprinkle each pizza with the onion, bell pepper, pineapple, and jalapeño.

3. Distribute dollops of chickpea spread evenly over each pizza. If desired, sprinkle with chopped Tofurky.

4. Bake for 15 minutes, or until the crusts are lightly golden. Serve warm. Store leftovers in an airtight container in the refrigerator for up to 1 week.

Substitute it: Use pita or naan bread to make individual-size pizzas. You can also use 9-inch whole-grain tortillas or homemade tortillas (page 106) to make this recipe lower in sodium, or use Engine 2 brand's whole-wheat pizza crusts for another store-bought option.

Per serving: Calories: 293; Total Fat: 9g; Saturated Fat: 3g; Cholesterol: 0mg; Sodium: 245mg; Carbohydrates: 51g; Fiber: 6g; Total Sugar: 19g; Added Sugar: 0g; Protein: 8g; Potassium: 606mg; Magnesium: 43mg; Vitamin K: 9mcg

Easy Zucchini-lini and "Meat" Sauce

5 Ingredients or Fewer, 30 Minutes or Less, Extra-Low Sodium, Gluten-Free
Serves 4 / Prep time: 10 minutes / Cook time: 20 minutes

Instead of getting a stomachache and wanting to take a nap from eating too much spaghetti, pile that plate high and feel energized and alive. This meal replaces some of the spaghetti with zucchini-lini (zucchini noodles), so you can feel satisfied and fuller for longer and benefit from more micronutrients.

6 ounces whole-grain spaghetti or fettuc-cine noodles

½ cup red lentils, rinsed

1 (24-ounce) jar reduced-sodium or no-salt-added marinara

2 medium zucchini, spiralized or peeled into long thin strips

½ cup Three-Seed "Parmesan" (optional; page 135)

1. In a large pot, cook the pasta according to the package directions.

2. Meanwhile, in a medium saucepan, combine the red lentils and marinara and bring to a boil over high heat. Reduce the heat to medium and simmer for 15 to 20 minutes, stirring frequently, until the lentils are cooked and soft.

3. Place the zucchini noodles in a colander or sieve set in the sink. Drain the pasta over the zucchini noodles. Transfer the pasta and zucchini back into the large pot and toss to combine.

4. Divide the pasta and zucchini-lini evenly among four bowls. Top with lentil sauce. If desired, garnish each bowl with 2 tablespoons "parmesan."

5. Serve warm. Store leftovers in an airtight container in the refrigerator for up to 1 week.

Make it easier: You can buy a little handheld spiralizer for about $10 online to make noodles out of zucchini. If you don't have one, make thick long noodles with a potato peeler. This is also fun to do with carrots and cucumber.

Substitute it: Instead of Three-Seed "Parmesan," just sprinkle 1 tablespoon of nutritional yeast and 1 tablespoon of hemp seeds or chopped raw walnuts on top of each bowl before serving.

Per serving: Calories: 339; Total Fat: 5g; Saturated Fat: 1g; Cholesterol: 0mg; Sodium: 61mg; Carbohydrates: 63g; Fiber: 10g; Total Sugar: 13g; Added Sugar: 0g; Protein: 15g; Potassium: 1,154mg; Magnesium: 62mg; Vitamin K: 28mcg

Spaghetti Squash Marinara

5 Ingredients or Fewer, Extra-Low Sodium, Gluten-Free
Serves 4 / Prep time: 10 minutes / Cook time: 25 minutes

Spaghetti squash is such a fun alternative to traditional spaghetti. And even though it looks and tastes impressive, it is definitely not difficult to make. Just be sure to purchase a marinara sauce that is labeled "reduced-sodium" or "no-salt-added" with less than 300mg of sodium per serving, and try to find one without added oil. I like the Trader Giotto's organic no-salt-added marinara from Trader Joe's.

1 medium spaghetti squash

2 cups reduced-sodium or no-salt-added marinara sauce, divided

2 cups chopped mushrooms

2 cups chopped spinach

1 (15-ounce) can no-salt-added cannellini beans, drained and rinsed (or 1½ cups home-cooked)

1. Preheat the oven to 400°F.

2. Using a large heavy knife, slice the squash in half lengthwise. Remove the seeds and place both halves cut-side down on a rimmed baking sheet. Bake for about 25 minutes, or until easily pierced with a fork.

3. Meanwhile, in a medium saucepan, combine ½ cup marinara, the mushrooms, and spinach and cook over medium-high heat for 5 to 10 minutes, until the mushrooms are tender and the spinach is wilted.

4. Once the spaghetti squash is done, scrape the strands into the saucepan. Add the remaining 1½ cups marinara and the beans and mix well to combine.

5. Divide into four servings and serve warm. Store leftovers in an airtight container in the refrigerator for up to 1 week.

Flavor boost: Add garlic, onion, and herbs (like basil, thyme, oregano, and sage) or a salt-free Italian seasoning blend to the sauce. Serve topped with Three-Seed "Parmesan" (page 135).

Per serving: Calories: 362; Total Fat: 3g; Saturated Fat: 0g; Cholesterol: 0mg; Sodium: 118mg; Carbohydrates: 70g; Fiber: 18g; Total Sugar: 15g; Added Sugar: 0g; Protein: 18g; Potassium: 1,129mg; Magnesium: 101mg; Vitamin K: 84mcg

Simple Stir-Fry

30 Minutes or Less, Gluten-Free, One-Pot
Serves 4 / Prep time: 10 minutes / Cook time: 20 minutes

Hate throwing food away? Me, too. I love trying new recipes and, without fail, by the end of the week there are always random leftover vegetables and grains that didn't make it into the meals. This simple stir-fry was, and still is, a solid weekly staple for cleaning out the refrigerator before making a grocery store run.

4 garlic cloves, minced, or 1 tablespoon minced fresh ginger

¼ cup water

4 cups roughly chopped mixed green vegetables (beets, broccoli, Brussels sprouts, asparagus, celery)

1 cup roughly chopped mushrooms

8 large kale, collard, or bok choy leaves, roughly chopped

3 cups cooked brown rice or quinoa

1 (15-ounce) can no-salt-added black beans, pinto beans, or kidney beans, drained and rinsed

2 tablespoons coconut aminos or reduced-sodium tamari

½ cup crushed raw peanuts, walnuts, or pumpkin seeds

2 teaspoons red pepper flakes

1. In a large skillet, combine the garlic or ginger and water and heat over medium-high heat.

2. Add the sturdier veggies (like beets, broccoli, Brussels sprouts) first and cook for 5 to 10 minutes. Add the mushrooms and cook for 3 more minutes. Add the leafy greens last and cook until wilted, about 5 more minutes. Continue to add water as needed and cook until the water is evaporated.

3. Reduce the heat and stir in the cooked rice, beans, and coconut aminos. Mix well to combine and remove from the heat.

4. Serve warm, topped with nuts or seeds and pepper flakes. Store leftovers in an airtight container in the refrigerator for up to 1 week.

Substitute it: Try a cubed block of tempeh instead of beans and stir in 2 tablespoons of unsalted, unsweetened creamy peanut butter for a creamy peanut-y stir-fry.

Per serving: Calories: 424; Total Fat: 12g; Saturated Fat: 2g; Cholesterol: 0mg; Sodium: 205mg; Carbohydrates: 67g; Fiber: 14g; Total Sugar: 3g; Added Sugar: 0g; Protein: 16g; Potassium: 885mg; Magnesium: 146mg; Vitamin K: 193mcg

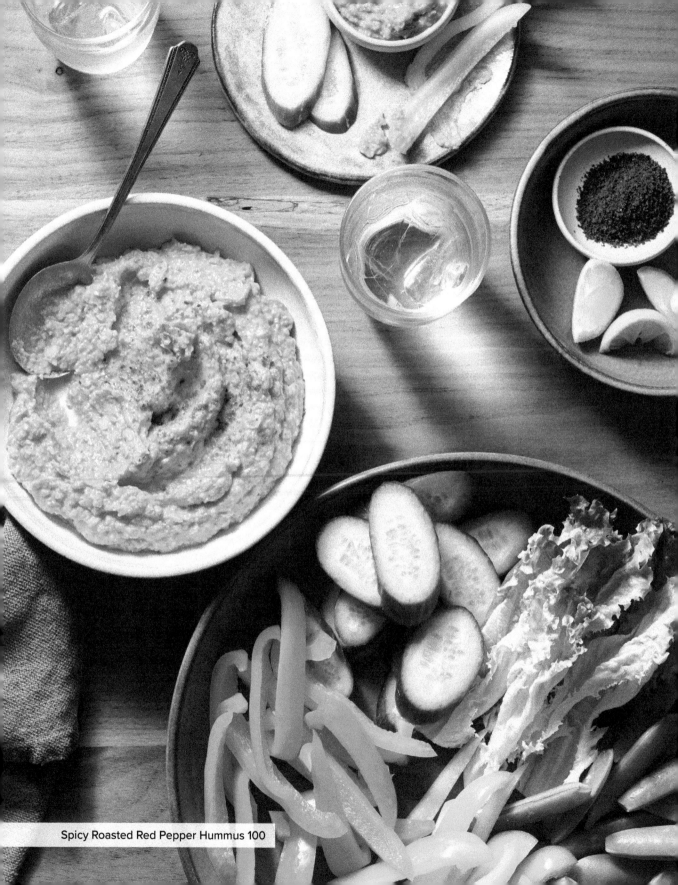

Spicy Roasted Red Pepper Hummus 100

Sides and Snacks

Spicy Roasted Chickpeas

5 Ingredients or Fewer, Extra-Low Sodium, Gluten-Free
Serves 4 / Prep time: 5 minutes / Cook time: 30 minutes

Everyone can use a little extra spice and crunch in their life—plus some plant-based protein, iron, and fiber. Reach for these as a snack, stuff into sandwiches, sizzle with stir-fries, serve on a salad—these Spicy Roasted Chickpeas make everything taste better.

1 (15.5-ounce) can no-salt-added chickpeas, drained, plus 1 tablespoon reserved chickpea liquid (aquafaba)

½ tablespoon ground cumin

½ tablespoon smoked paprika

1 teaspoon garlic powder

Pinch freshly ground black pepper

1. Preheat the oven to 425°F. Line a rimmed baking sheet with parchment paper.

2. Spread the chickpeas onto the baking sheet and bake for 15 minutes, or until dry.

3. Meanwhile, in a large bowl, mix the aquafaba with the cumin, paprika, garlic powder, and black pepper.

4. Remove the chickpeas from the oven. Leave the oven on. Transfer the chickpeas to the bowl and mix to coat well with the spices.

5. Spread them on the baking sheet again and bake for another 15 minutes, or until crispy.

6. Serve warm or store leftovers in an airtight container at room temperature for up to 1 week.

Flavor boost: For an extra kick, add ¼ teaspoon of cayenne pepper to the spice mix. The chickpeas may lose their crispness after a day or so. To retain flavor and texture, reheat them for 5 to 10 minutes in the oven before serving.

Substitute it: Use this mixture of spices to make roasted sweet potatoes or sweet potato fries by using sliced potatoes instead of chickpeas. They may need to cook a little longer depending on the size of the slices.

Per serving: Calories: 86; Total Fat: 2g; Saturated Fat: 0g; Cholesterol: 0mg; Sodium: 123mg; Carbohydrates: 14g; Fiber: 4g; Total Sugar: 2g; Added Sugar: 0g; Protein: 4g; Potassium: 86mg; Magnesium: 18mg; Vitamin K: 2mcg

Spicy Roasted Red Pepper Hummus

30 Minutes or Less, Gluten-Free, One-Pot
Serves 8 / Prep time: 15 minutes

Studies show that adding fresh lemon juice to plant sources of iron can help boost iron absorption by 67 percent. The vitamin C acts as a co-factor to help absorb plant-based iron. This is why fresh hummus, with a lemon juice/chickpea combo, is absolutely an essential staple on a plant-based diet. I like Siete brand hot sauce for this recipe.

2 (15-ounce) cans no-salt-added chickpeas, drained and rinsed

⅓ cup jarred roasted red peppers

2 garlic cloves, peeled

5 tablespoons hot sauce

2 tablespoons tahini

2 tablespoons apple cider vinegar

1 teaspoon smoked paprika

Juice of ½ lemon

1. In a food processor, combine the chickpeas, roasted peppers, garlic, hot sauce, tahini, vinegar, smoked paprika, and lemon juice and process for 1 to 2 minutes, until smooth.

2. Store in an airtight container in the refrigerator for up to 1 week.

Flavor boost: Serve with raw veggies, in wraps or sandwiches, on salad bowls, or atop Five-Ingredient Beet Burgers (page 72). There is also nothing better than a rainbow hummus appetizer platter at any gathering: On a giant cutting board, lay out this hummus along with Beet Spread (page 139) and Health-Nut Cacao Spread (page 134), plus celery, carrots, broccoli, cauliflower, grapes, cherry tomatoes, and every color of sweet bell pepper.

Per serving: Calories: 107; Total Fat: 4g; Saturated Fat: 0g; Cholesterol: 0mg; Sodium: 248mg; Carbohydrates: 15g; Fiber: 4g; Total Sugar: 2g; Added Sugar: 0g; Protein: 5g; Potassium: 89mg; Magnesium: 19mg; Vitamin K: 2mcg

Baked Chips

5 Ingredients or Fewer, 30 Minutes or Less, Extra-Low Sodium, One-Pot
Serves 3 / Prep time: 5 minutes / Cook time: 18 minutes

The tortilla chips that we buy in the store have been scientifically designed to make us crave more. These chips, while delicious, are not here to mess with your head or increase your heart disease risk. When buying flour tortillas, focus on those made with whole-grain flour, with less than 200mg of sodium per serving, preferably no oil, and as few ingredients and additives as possible. Also, the thinner the tortilla, the better for making chips.

4 (9-inch) whole-grain flour tortillas, homemade (page 106) or store-bought

1. Preheat the oven to 425°F.

2. Cut the tortillas into 6 triangles each and spread evenly onto baking sheets, with no overlapping.

3. Bake for 15 to 18 minutes, until the chips are perfectly golden and crispy. Store the chips in an airtight container at room temperature for up to 1 week.

Flavor boost: Before baking, with your finger or a pastry brush, brush each chip lightly with low-sodium vegetable broth or pickle juice, and dust the chips with garlic powder, paprika, cayenne, or whatever spices and herbs you like.

Per serving: Calories: 136; Total Fat: 1g; Saturated Fat: 0g; Cholesterol: 0mg; Sodium: 0mg; Carbohydrates: 28g; Fiber: 4g; Total Sugar: 0g; Added Sugar: 0g; Protein: 5g; Potassium: 144mg; Magnesium: 219mg; Vitamin K: 0mg

Arame Tahini-Ginger Coleslaw

30 Minutes or Less, Gluten-Free
Serves 8 / Prep time: 15 minutes

Arame is a is dense in micronutrients including iodine. Cabbage contains polysterols, which have a similar structure to cholesterol and have been shown to help lower LDL cholesterol.

1 cup lightly packed dried arame

3 tablespoons tahini

Juice of ½ lime

2 tablespoons apple cider vinegar

1 tablespoon coconut aminos or reduced-sodium tamari

1½ tablespoons minced peeled fresh ginger

½ tablespoon maple syrup

8 cups thinly sliced red or green cabbage

2 cups grated carrots

1 cup chopped fresh cilantro

1. Rinse the dried arame in cool water and drain. In a medium bowl, submerge the rinsed arame in water and let soak while preparing the other ingredients.

2. In a small bowl, mix together the tahini, lime juice, vinegar, coconut aminos, ginger, and maple syrup. Set the dressing aside.

3. Drain the arame and transfer to a large bowl. Add the cabbage, carrots, and cilantro. Mix the dressing into the cabbage mixture.

4. Serve, or chill before serving. Store leftovers in an airtight container in the refrigerator for up to 1 week.

Per serving: Calories: 124; Total Fat: 0g; Saturated Fat: 0g; Cholesterol: 0mg; Sodium: 313mg; Carbohydrates: 23g; Fiber: 7g; Total Sugar: 10g; Added Sugar: 1.5g; Protein: 5g; Potassium: 971mg; Magnesium: 60mg; Vitamin K: 79mcg

Celery and Cinnamon Apple Plate

5 Ingredients or Fewer, 30 Minutes or Less, Extra-Low Sodium, Gluten-Free, One-Pot

Serves 2 / Prep time: 10 minutes

When I was growing up, my favorite snack was my mom's cinnamon apple plate. She would slice the apple into perfect little wedges and dust each with cinnamon and I think a little sugar, too. This is my not-so-grown-up spin on the old classic.

1 apple

2 tablespoons unsalted, unsweetened peanut butter

3 celery stalks, finely diced

¼ cup raisins

½ teaspoon ground cinnamon

1. Slice the apples horizontally into thin chip-like rounds and remove the seeds. The slices should have a beautiful star shape in the center.

2. On a large plate or two small plates, layer the apple rounds on the bottom. Spread a little peanut butter on some of them and sprinkle the plate with diced celery, raisins, and cinnamon.

3. Enjoy immediately.

Substitute it: Try chopped walnuts, hemp seeds, or Health-Nut Cacao Spread (page 134) instead of the peanut butter. Celery and Health-Nut Cacao Spread is one of my all-time favorite combos.

Per serving: Calories: 207; Total Fat: 9g; Saturated Fat: 2g; Cholesterol: 0mg; Sodium: 56mg; Carbohydrates: 33g; Fiber: 5g; Total Sugar: 2g; Added Sugar: 1g; Protein: 5g; Potassium: 480mg; Magnesium: 45mg; Vitamin K: 20mcg

Perfect Corn Bread

30 Minutes or Less, Extra-Low Sodium
Serves 12 / Prep time: 10 minutes / Cook time: 20 minutes

This lighter and healthier version of corn bread pairs well with every meal. It will have your guests saying, "Who needs an entree? I just want more corn bread!"

1 cup corn flour or cornmeal

¾ cup whole-wheat flour

1 tablespoon baking powder

1 cup unsweetened plain soy milk

¼ cup mashed avocado

1 teaspoon apple cider vinegar

¼ teaspoon grated lemon zest

1 teaspoon fresh lemon juice

1. Preheat the oven to 400°F. Line an 8-by-8-inch square baking pan with parchment paper and set aside.

2. In a large bowl, combine the corn flour, whole-wheat flour, and baking powder.

3. In a medium bowl, stir together the milk, avocado, vinegar, lemon zest, and lemon juice. Pour the wet ingredients into the dry ingredients and gently mix until just combined.

4. Scrape the batter into the prepared baking pan and smooth the top with a rubber spatula.

5. Bake for 20 minutes, or until cracks form and a knife comes out clean. Serve warm.

6. To store leftovers, allow to cool for at least 20 minutes. Store in an airtight container on the counter for up to 1 week.

Substitute it: Instead of whole-wheat flour, use gluten-free baking flour, oat flour, rice flour, or all-purpose flour. Instead of mashed avocado, use mashed banana or applesauce.

Flavor boost: For a sweeter corn bread, add 2 tablespoons of maple syrup or Truvia granulated sweetener or 2 dropperfuls of liquid stevia extract. I love the brightness that lemon juice and lemon zest provide. Try doubling the amount of lemon juice and lemon zest and see how you like it.

Per serving: Calories: 77; Total Fat: 2g; Saturated Fat: 0g; Cholesterol: 0mg; Sodium: 132mg; Carbohydrates: 14g; Fiber: 2g; Total Sugar: 0g; Added Sugar: 0g; Protein: 3g; Potassium: 84mg; Magnesium: 18mg; Vitamin K: 1mcg

Homemade Flour Tortillas

5 Ingredients or Fewer, Extra-Low Sodium
Makes 8 tortillas / Prep time: 20 minutes / Cook time: 20 minutes

Can't find a tortilla that doesn't have unwanted added ingredients? Neither can I, which is why I make my own. Homemade tortillas—sounds impressive doesn't it? Put the flour that's been sitting around in your cupboard to good use and have fun wowing your friends and family with how effortlessly you whip these up. Don't have a rolling pin? Use a can of beans, a jar, or any other cylinder you've got.

2 cups whole-wheat flour, plus more for rolling

⅔ cup water

1. In a large bowl, combine the flour and water. Then, using your clean hands, knead and fold to mix the water and flour so it forms a ball of dough that's not sticky and is easy to pick up.

2. Put the ball of dough on a floured cutting board and, using a large sharp knife, divide it in half, then divide those two pieces in half again. Repeat one more time, so you have 8 pieces of dough. Roll each piece of dough into a ball and set aside.

3. Lightly flour a rolling pin and the cutting board again. Then roll one of the 8 pieces of dough into a round. Make it as thin as possible without ripping it or making it impossible to move.

4. Heat a medium skillet over medium heat and transfer the dough round onto the hot pan. Cook the dough for 2 to 3 minutes on each side, until the dough rises off the pan slightly and the edges

become golden brown. Repeat the process to make any additional tortillas that are going to be eaten right away.

5. Store the rest of the balls of dough in an airtight container in the refrigerator to be used through-out the week, or cook the tortillas ahead of time and store them in an airtight container in the refrigerator to be toasted or reheated in a pan for future use.

Substitute it: For lighter tasting, more authentic tortillas, use all-purpose flour instead of whole-wheat flour. Or try them with gluten-free all-purpose flour or even chickpea flour. Whatever flour you like or happen to have is worth a try.

Flavor boost: In a high-powered blender, blend the water (that will be mixed with the flour) with a handful of spinach, kale, ¼ small beet, or even some fresh herbs you may have in the refrigerator to make spinach, kale, beet, or herb tortillas.

Per serving (1 tortilla): Calories: 102; Total Fat: 1g; Saturated Fat: 0g; Cholesterol: 0mg; Sodium: 0mg; Carbohydrates: 21g; Fiber: 3g; Total Sugar: 0g; Added Sugar: 0g; Protein: 4g; Potassium: 108mg; Magnesium: 164mg; Vitamin K: 0mcg

Maple-Balsamic Roasted Veggies

5 Ingredients or Fewer, Extra-Low Sodium, Gluten-Free
Serves 6 / Prep time: 10 minutes / Cook time: 35 minutes

This veggie side dish pairs well with nearly every main-course meal. I like a combinations of red bell pepper, zucchini, broccoli, mushrooms, and onions, but use whatever vegetables you prefer or have.

3 tablespoons balsamic vinegar

2 tablespoons maple syrup

3 garlic cloves, minced

¼ cup tahini

6 cups chopped vegetables of choice

1. Preheat the oven to 375°F. Line two rimmed baking sheets with parchment paper. Set aside.

2. In a large bowl, whisk together the balsamic vinegar, maple syrup, garlic, and tahini. Add the vegetables and mix until they are well coated.

3. Spread the vegetables evenly over the baking sheets and bake for 25 to 35 minutes, until the vegetables are fork-tender.

4. Serve warm. Store leftovers in an airtight container in the refrigerator for up to 1 week.

Substitute it: Use orange juice instead of maple syrup or reduced-sodium tamari instead of balsamic vinegar.

Per serving: Calories: 110; Total Fat: 6g; Saturated Fat: 1g; Cholesterol: 0mg; Sodium: 38mg; Carbohydrates: 13g; Fiber: 3g; Total Sugar: 7g; Added Sugar: 4g; Protein: 4g; Potassium: 295mg; Magnesium: 27mg; Vitamin K: 72mcg

Easy Microwave-Baked Stuffed Sweet Potato

5 Ingredients or Fewer, 30 Minutes or Less, Extra-Low Sodium, Gluten-Free, One-Pot

Serves 1 / Prep time: 5 minutes / Cook time: 10 minutes

Sweet potatoes should be on every list of "foods for longevity." Why? In Okinawa, Japan, known to have the most people in a region to live over 100 and to have the highest life expectancy for its people, the population consumes 85 percent of its calories from carbohydrates and about 60 percent of its calories from, you guessed it, sweet potatoes.

1 medium organic sweet potato

2 tablespoons chopped raw walnuts

Ground cinnamon

1. Pierce the potato 5 to 10 times with a knife or fork.

2. Place the potato in a microwave-safe medium bowl and cover with a microwave-safe lid or plate. Cook for 5 minutes, check tenderness, flip, and cook for another 2 to 5 minutes, or until tender and easily pierced with a fork.

3. Slice in half, stuff with walnuts and cinnamon to taste, and serve warm. Store leftovers in an airtight container in the refrigerator for up to 1 week.

Flavor boost: Instead of walnuts, try another nut, seed, or nut butter you like. Baked sweet potatoes are also delicious with other toppings and seasonings, from pomegranate and cacao powder to Lemon-Tahini Dressing (page 141), parsley, and garlic powder.

Per serving: Calories: 208; Total Fat: 10g; Saturated Fat: 1g; Cholesterol: 0mg; Sodium: 72mg; Carbohydrates: 28g; Fiber: 5g; Total Sugar: 6g; Added Sugar: 0g; Protein: 4g; Potassium: 504mg; Magnesium: 56mg; Vitamin K: 3mcg

Miso-Ginger Brussels Sprouts

30 Minutes or Less, Gluten-Free
Serves 4 / Prep time: 10 minutes / Cook time: 20 minutes

The first time I made this recipe, I sat down and ate all the Brussels sprouts myself. I just couldn't stop; they are so good. This is a perfect side dish for Lemon and Herb Tofu Fillets (page 84) or any holiday meal. It's also a great addition to potlucks.

1 pound Brussels sprouts, halved

⅓ cup water

2 tablespoons sweet white miso paste

1 tablespoon maple syrup

1 teaspoon Dijon mustard

1 tablespoon grated fresh ginger

1 tablespoon apple cider vinegar

2 tablespoons tahini

1. Preheat the oven to 400°F. Line a rimmed baking sheet with parchment paper and set aside.

2. In a large skillet, water-sauté (see page 18) the Brussels sprouts over medium-high heat in the water for 8 to 10 minutes. Stir occasionally and add water, 2 tablespoons at a time, if necessary to prevent sticking. Once the water has evaporated, remove from the heat.

3. In a medium bowl, combine the miso, maple syrup, mustard, ginger, vinegar, and tahini and mix well.

4. Pour the mixture over the sprouts in the skillet and stir well to combine. Transfer the sprouts to the baking sheet, being sure to get all the sauce. Spread evenly on the baking sheet and bake for about 10 minutes, or until fork-tender.

5. Serve warm. Store leftovers in an airtight container in the refrigerator for up to 1 week.

Substitute it: If you don't want to use maple syrup, feel free to blend the miso, mustard, ginger, vinegar, and tahini in a high-powered blender with 2 pitted dates and 1 to 2 tablespoons of simmering water. This recipe is also delicious with broccoli, parsnips, asparagus, and even sliced cabbage.

Per serving: Calories: 127; Total Fat: 5g; Saturated Fat: 1g; Cholesterol: 0mg; Sodium: 338mg; Carbohydrates: 19g; Fiber: 7g; Total Sugar: 7g; Added Sugar: 3g; Protein: 7g; Potassium: 509mg; Magnesium: 37mg; Vitamin K: 201mcg

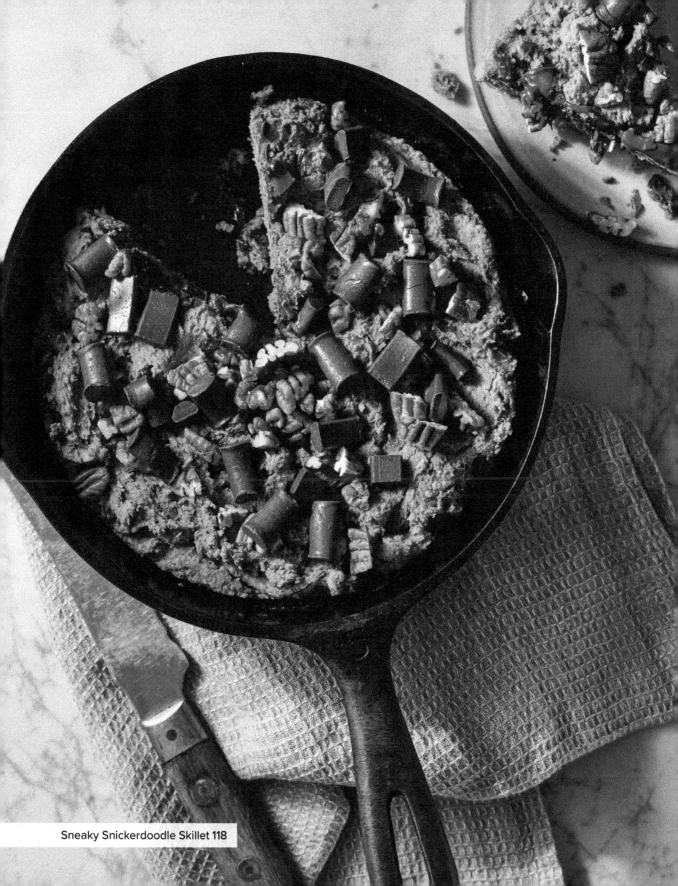

Sneaky Snickerdoodle Skillet 118

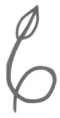

Sweet Treats

Five-Ingredient Frozen Yogurt Bars

5 Ingredients or Fewer, Extra-Low Sodium
Makes 12 yogurt bars / Prep time: 5 minutes, plus 1 hour to chill

These are a sweet, refreshing energy boost that may keep you from getting hungry and irritable because 90 percent of serotonin, the body's "feel-good" neurotransmitter, gets produced in our gastrointestinal tract. Nothing promotes the growth of beneficial microbiota better than fermented foods like yogurt and a diet rich in a diversity of plants.

1 cup rolled oats

1 cup pitted Medjool dates

⅓ cup unsalted, unsweetened almond butter

½ teaspoon vanilla extract

1 cup store-bought unsweetened vanilla plant-based yogurt or Fresh Walnut Yogurt (page 144)

1. Line an 8-by-8-inch baking pan with parchment paper and set aside.

2. In a food processor, blend the oats for about 30 seconds. Add the dates, almond butter, and vanilla and pulse for another minute or so, scraping down the sides frequently, until well combined. The mixture should be very thick and chunky, not smooth.

3. Spread the bar mixture evenly into the lined pan and press firmly so the top is smooth.

4. With a rubber spatula, spread the yogurt over the top. Freeze for at least 1 hour or overnight.

5. Divide into 12 bars and serve chilled, or keep in the freezer in an airtight container for up to 2 weeks.

Flavor boost: Garnish with optional toppings like pomegranate seeds, hemp seeds, chopped raw walnuts, sliced bananas, cacao nibs, toasted coconut, or frozen wild blueberries.

Per serving (1 bar): Calories: 97; Total Fat: 5g; Saturated Fat: 1g; Cholesterol: 0mg; Sodium: 7mg; Carbohydrates: 11g; Fiber: 0g; Total Sugar: 5g; Added Sugar: 0g; Protein: 3g; Potassium: 133mg; Magnesium: 32mg; Vitamin K: 0.23mcg

Chocolate "Nice-Cream" Sundaes

5 Ingredients or Fewer, 30 Minutes or Less, Extra-Low Sodium, Gluten-Free, One-Pot

Serves 4 / Prep time: 10 minutes

Did you know that potassium increases the release of nitric oxide, the magic compound that opens up our blood vessels? Eating a single high-potassium meal can improve arterial function, whereas eating a high-sodium meal can impair arterial function within 30 minutes. Get plenty of heart-disease healing potassium with ice cream? Oh yes, life is good.

4 ripe bananas, cut into chunks and frozen

2 teaspoons vanilla extract

¼ cup cacao powder

½ cup walnuts

1 cup fresh or frozen berries

1. In a high-powered blender or food processor, blend the bananas, vanilla, and cacao powder until smooth.

2. Assemble each sundae with one-quarter of the nice cream mixture, 2 tablespoons walnuts, and ¼ cup fresh berries. Serve immediately.

Flavor tip: It *does matter* how ripe the bananas are. If not ripe enough, the sundaes will taste off. Wait for bananas to have a few brown spots before freezing.

Make it easier: This recipe requires a very high-quality blender, like a Vitamix or NutriBullet, or a food processor. Scared you're going to break your food processor? Add unsweetened vanilla soy milk, 1 tablespoon at a time, to help or let the frozen bananas sit out for 5 to 10 minutes to thaw a little bit before blending.

Per serving: Calories: 256.2; Total Fat: 11g; Saturated Fat: 1g; Cholesterol: 0mg; Sodium: 2mg; Carbohydrates: 39g; Fiber: 8g; Total Sugar: 20g; Added Sugar: 0g; Protein: 5g; Potassium: 621mg; Magnesium: 58mg; Vitamin K: 10mcg

Super Mint–Chocolate Chip Soft Serve

30 Minutes or Less, Extra-Low Sodium, Gluten-Free, One-Pot
Serves 4 / Prep time: 10 minutes

Finally: a dessert that loves you just as much as you love it. This soft-serve "nice cream" helps build blood with plant-based iron from the spinach. And did you know that 1 cup of spinach has about twice as much potassium as a large banana? Dreams do come true: ice cream with endless benefits. I like Lily's brand chocolate chunks.

½ cup packed spinach	2 teaspoons vanilla extract
¼ cup packed fresh mint leaves	4 ripe bananas, cut into chunks and frozen
¼ cup unsweetened vanilla soy milk	¼ cup vegan dark chocolate chunks

1. In a high-powered blender or food processor, blend the spinach, mint leaves, soy milk, and vanilla for 1 to 2 minutes, until very smooth, scraping down the sides as needed.

2. Add the bananas and blend until smooth. Pulse in the dark chocolate chunks and serve immediately.

Flavor boost: Want a hit of caffeine and antioxidants? Try adding 2 teaspoons of matcha green tea powder. It's like a sweet iced matcha latte in a perfectly smooth soft-serve form. Enjoy!

Per serving: Calories: 180; Total Fat: 4g; Saturated Fat: 2g; Cholesterol: 0mg; Sodium: 28mg; Carbohydrates: 34g; Fiber: 4g; Total Sugar: 17g; Added Sugar: 2g; Protein: 6g; Potassium: 544mg; Magnesium: 38mg; Vitamin K: 19mcg

Sneaky Snickerdoodle Skillet

30 Minutes or Less, Gluten-Free

Serves 6 / Prep time: 10 minutes / Cook time: 20 minutes

This skillet is called "sneaky" because the base of the dough is beans. White beans contain resistant starch, which has been shown to prevent blood sugar spikes. One cup of white beans has about 20 percent of the recommended daily intake for potassium. In a study of about 250,000 people, researchers found that increasing potassium by 1,640mg per day decreased stroke risk by 21 percent. White beans are also a great source of fiber (about 17 grams per cup, or 75 percent of the recommended daily intake) and plant-based protein.

Coconut or avocado oil cooking spray

½ cup tightly packed pitted Medjool dates

1 ripe banana

1½ teaspoons ground cinnamon

¼ cup unsalted, unsweetened peanut butter

1½ tablespoons unsweetened plain soy milk

2 teaspoons vanilla extract

1 (15-ounce) can no-salt-added white beans, drained and rinsed

½ cup gluten-free all-purpose flour or oat flour

2 teaspoons baking powder

⅓ cup vegan dark chocolate chunks (70-percent cacao or higher)

⅓ cup chopped raw pecans (optional)

1. Preheat the oven to 350°F. Mist a cast-iron skillet or cake pan with cooking spray. If you're using a cake pan, you can line it with a round of parchment paper instead of using the oil spray. Set aside.

2. In a food processor, blend the dates, banana, cinnamon, peanut butter, soy milk, and vanilla for 2 to 3 minutes, until smooth. Add the white beans and process for another 2 minutes, or until smooth,

occasionally scraping down the sides with a rubber spatula.

3. With the machine running, add the flour 1 tablespoon at a time. Add the baking powder and blend for about 10 more seconds.

4. Take out the processor blade and fold in half of the chocolate chunks and pecans (if using). Spread the mixture evenly in the skillet or pan. Top with the rest of the chocolate chunks and pecans.

5. Bake for 20 minutes, or until golden, Serve warm. Store leftovers in an airtight container for up to 1 week.

Per serving: Calories: 322; Total Fat: 12g; Saturated Fat: 5g; Cholesterol: 0mg; Sodium: 392mg; Carbohydrates: 48g; Fiber: 8g; Total Sugar: 8g; Added Sugar: 5g; Protein: 9g; Potassium: 616mg; Magnesium: 63mg; Vitamin K: 3mcg

Simple Lemon Cookies

5 Ingredients or Fewer, Extra-Low Sodium, Gluten-Free
Makes 12 cookies / Prep time: 10 minutes,
plus 10 minutes to chill / Cook time: 18 minutes

Brew a pot of chamomile tea, take a deep breath, and say hello to the perfect combination of tart, sweet, and simply divine with these lemon cookies. Don't want to use maple syrup? Replace the maple syrup with ¼ cup of unsweetened vanilla soy milk plus 28 drops of stevia extract. Or, try using 4 pitted Medjool dates simmered in 2 tablespoons of water for 10 minutes and blended until smooth.

¼ cup maple syrup

1 teaspoon grated lemon zest

⅓ cup fresh lemon juice (about 2 lemons)

1 teaspoon vanilla extract

1 cup almond flour

1. Preheat the oven to 350°F. Line a rimmed baking sheet with parchment paper. Set aside.

2. In a medium bowl, mix together the maple syrup, lemon zest, lemon juice, and vanilla. Stir in the almond flour, about ¼ cup at a time. The cookie batter should be sticky and thick, not dry and crumbly.

3. Place the dough in the refrigerator for 5 to 10 minutes to set.

4. Using a tablespoon, scoop out 12 rounded scoops. Form each into a ball and place it on the baking sheet. With the back of a wet fork, score the cookies vertically and horizontally.

5. Bake for 15 to 18 minutes, until golden and crispy around the edges. Let the cookies cool on the baking sheet for another 5 to 10 minutes before enjoying.

6. Be sure the cookies are completely cooled before storing in an airtight container in a cool, dry place for up to 1 week.

Per serving (1 cookie): Calories: 73; Total Fat: 5g; Saturated Fat: 0g; Cholesterol: 0mg; Sodium: 2mg; Carbohydrates: 7g; Fiber: 1g; Total Sugar: 5g; Added Sugar: 4g; Protein: 2g; Potassium: 91mg; Magnesium: 26mg; Vitamin K: 0mcg

Ginger-Tahini Tea Cookies

5 Ingredients or Fewer, 30 Minutes or Less, Extra-Low Sodium, Gluten-Free
Makes 18 cookies / Prep time: 10 minutes,
plus 5 minutes to chill / Cook time: 15 minutes

These sweet little cookies are quite potent powerhouses of warming vanilla-gingery flavor, and the perfect chew-to-crunch ratio—designed for refined and sophisticated herbal tea sippers.

½ cup packed pitted Medjool dates

¼ cup hot water

¾ cup tahini

2 teaspoons grated fresh ginger

2 teaspoons vanilla extract

2 cups almond flour

1. Preheat the oven to 350°F. Line a rimmed baking sheet with parchment paper. Set aside.

2. Meanwhile, in a bowl, soak the dates in the hot water for about 5 minutes to soften.

3. In a food processor, combine the dates and their soaking water, the tahini, ginger, and vanilla and blend until smooth.

4. With the machine running, add the almond meal, ¼ cup at a time, until the dough is not sticky, wet, or crumbly.

5. Transfer the dough to the freezer for 5 minutes to set.

6. Scoop out rounded tablespoons of dough and form into balls. Place on the baking sheet. Then, with a wet fork, press to score the cookies vertically and horizontally.

7. Bake for 13 to 15 minutes, until perfectly golden to light brown, not dark brown. Cool for 5 to 7 minutes on the baking sheet.

8. Enjoy warm. Store leftover cookies in an airtight container in a cool, dry place for up to 1 week or in the freezer for up to 2 weeks.

Substitute it: Use 2 teaspoons of ground ginger instead of grated fresh ginger. Also, instead of dates, use ⅓ to ½ cup of maple syrup and mix the dough by hand in a bowl instead of in a food processor.

Per serving (1 cookie): Calories: 144; Total Fat: 12g; Saturated Fat: 1g; Cholesterol: 0mg; Sodium: 16mg; Carbohydrates: 8g; Fiber: 3g; Total Sugar: 3g; Added Sugar: 0g; Protein: 5g; Potassium: 163mg; Magnesium: 47mg; Vitamin K: 0mcg

Peanut Butter Cookies

5 Ingredients or Fewer, 30 Minutes or Less, Extra-Low Sodium, Gluten-Free
Makes 18 cookies / Prep time: 15 minutes / Cook time: 15 minutes

I was the baby in the family with the sensitive stomach, and peanut butter cookies didn't used to sit right with me. It wasn't until after I was vegan for a few years that I reintroduced a veganized healthy version of peanut butter cookies into my life. 100 percent happiness, 0 percent stomachache.

¾ cup pitted Medjool dates

½ cup water

2 teaspoons baking powder

1 cup gluten-free all-purpose flour

1 cup unsalted, unsweetened peanut butter

2 ripe bananas

32 drops (2 full droppers) liquid stevia (optional)

1. Preheat the oven to 350°F. Line a rimmed baking sheet with parchment paper. Set aside.

2. Place the dates in a heatproof bowl. In a small saucepan, bring the water to a simmer, then pour over the dates. Cover and set aside for 2 to 5 minutes to soften.

3. In a large bowl, whisk together the baking powder and flour. Set aside.

4. In a food processor, blend the dates with their soaking water, the peanut butter, bananas, and stevia (if using) until very smooth, about 2 minutes.

5. Add the date mixture to the flour mixture and stir with a metal fork or spoon until just combined. Using an ice cream scoop or ¼-cup measuring cup, scoop the batter evenly into 18 cookies onto the baking sheet. With a wet fork, score the tops of the cookies vertically, then horizontally.

6. Bake for 15 minutes, or until risen and a slightly darker golden brown. Allow to cool for another 5 minutes before eating.

7. Serve warm. Store leftovers in an airtight container in a cool, dry place for up to 1 week.

Flavor boost: Not eating these fresh out of the oven? Put them in the toaster. They are much better warm! If these aren't sweet enough, experiment with adding the liquid stevia or use 1 to 2 tablespoons of liquid sweetener like maple syrup or agave.

Per serving (1 cookie): Calories: 230; Total Fat: 15g; Saturated Fat: 3g; Cholesterol: 0mg; Sodium: 62mg; Carbohydrates: 21g; Fiber: 3g; Total Sugar: 9g; Added Sugar: 2g; Protein: 7g; Potassium: 260mg; Magnesium: 55mg; Vitamin K: 0.32mcg

Raw Walnut Brownie Bites

30 Minutes or Less, Extra-Low Sodium, Gluten-Free
Makes 12 brownie bites / Prep time: 10 minutes, plus 20 minutes to chill

I keep this treat in my freezer for a chocolate fix or an energy boost. They're delicious dipped in Health-Nut Cacao Spread (page 134) or atop Super Mint–Chocolate Chip Soft Serve (page 117).

12 ounces raw walnuts (about 3 cups)	1½ teaspoons ground cinnamon
¾ cup tightly packed pitted Medjool dates	2 teaspoons vanilla extract
¼ cup cacao powder	1½ teaspoons fresh lemon juice

1. Line an 8-by-8-inch-inch baking pan with parchment paper. Set aside.

2. In a food processor, process the walnuts for 30 to 60 seconds, until a fine meal. Add the dates, cacao powder, cinnamon, vanilla, and lemon juice and blend for 2 minutes, or until well combined, scraping down the sides as needed.

3. Press the mixture firmly into the baking pan and let set in the freezer for 15 to 20 minutes.

4. Cut into 12 brownies and serve cold. Store leftovers in an airtight container in the refrigerator for up to 1 week or in the freezer for up to 2 weeks.

Per serving (1 brownie bite): Calories: 240; Total Fat: 14g; Saturated Fat: 1g; Cholesterol: 0mg; Sodium: 0mg; Carbohydrates: 29g; Fiber: 4g; Total Sugar: 23g; Added Sugar: 0g; Protein: 4g; Potassium: 257mg; Magnesium: 18mg; Vitamin K: 1mcg

Frozen Chocolate–Peanut Butter Banana Bites

5 Ingredients or Fewer, Extra-Low Sodium, Gluten-Free
Serves 6 / Prep time: 15 minutes, plus 2 hours to freeze

This frozen sweet treat requires only a few ingredients. I like Lily's brand chocolate chips sweetened with stevia for this recipe.

6 tablespoons unsalted, unsweetened peanut butter

3 ripe bananas, halved lengthwise and then crosswise (12 pieces)

6 tablespoons vegan dark chocolate chips

1. Line a large airtight container with parchment paper and set aside.

2. Spread 1 tablespoon peanut butter each on 6 banana pieces and press the remaining 6 pieces against the peanut butter to make a peanut butter sandwich.

3. In a small glass or metal bowl set over a pot of simmering water, melt the chocolate, stirring frequently. (Or microwave in a microwave-safe bowl in 30-second increments, stirring frequently, until able to drizzle.)

4. Drizzle the dark chocolate over the peanut butter-banana sandwiches. Freeze for at least 2 hours before serving. Store leftovers in an airtight container in the freezer for up to 1 month.

Per serving: Calories: 205; Total Fat: 13g; Saturated Fat: 4g; Cholesterol: 0mg; Sodium: 3mg; Carbohydrates: 25g; Fiber: 7g; Total Sugar: 9g; Added Sugar: 2g; Protein: 5g; Potassium: 392mg; Magnesium: 43mg; Vitamin K: 1mcg

Red Velvet Beet Brownies

30 Minutes or Less, Extra-Low Sodium, Gluten-Free
Makes 9 brownies / Prep time: 10 minutes / Cook time: 20 minutes

Who knew beets could be so good? While beets may have an earthy flavor, they also provide a unique sweetness that is simply divine when combined with chocolate. For how nutritious these ooey bites of perfection are, they're pretty out of this world.

15 to 20 pitted Medjool dates or ½ cup tightly packed regular dates

2½ cups finely chopped beets (about 2 medium)

½ tablespoon vanilla extract

1 teaspoon fresh lemon juice or apple cider vinegar

32 drops (2 full droppers) liquid stevia

¼ cup plus 2 tablespoons cacao powder

1¾ to 2½ cups oat flour

½ cup chopped raw walnuts (optional)

½ cup vegan dark chocolate chips (optional)

1. Preheat the oven to 375°F. Line an 8-by-8-inch baking pan with parchment paper. Set aside.

2. In a food processor, blend the dates, beets, vanilla, lemon juice, and stevia for 2 minutes, or until very smooth. Every 20 seconds or so, scrape down the sides with a rubber spatula to ensure it's well combined.

3. Add the cacao powder and blend. Add the oat flour, ¼ cup at a time, and blend until smooth and creamy. The batter should be sticky and spreadable, not super wet or dry.

4. Remove the processor blade and, if desired, fold in the walnuts and dark chocolate chips.

5. Spread the sticky and thick brownie batter evenly in the lined pan. Bake for 20 minutes, or until the color darkens and a knife inserted in the center comes out clean. Remove from the oven and allow to cool before cutting.

6. Cut into 9 brownies. Store leftovers in an airtight container in the refrigerator for up to 4 days.

Substitute it: Use all-purpose flour or gluten-free all-purpose flour instead of oat flour. Instead of the liquid stevia, use 1 to 2 tablespoons of liquid sweetener like maple syrup or agave or omit completely if desired.

Flavor boost: Make Murasaki sweet potato frosting to spread over these brownies by baking or steaming 1 medium Murasaki sweet potato until soft. (See Easy Microwave-Baked Sweet Potato, page 109, for the timing.) Peel the cooked potato and blend in a high-powered blender with 1½ cups of unsweetened vanilla soy milk, 1 teaspoon of vanilla extract, 1 to 2 teaspoons of lemon juice, and 1 dropper of liquid stevia. Blend for 1 minute, or until smooth and creamy. Spread over the brownies as a vanilla frosting.

Per serving (1 brownie): Calories: 260; Total Fat: 3g; Saturated Fat: 1g; Cholesterol: 0mg; Sodium: 11mg; Carbohydrates: 56g; Fiber: 8g; Total Sugar: 28g; Added Sugar: 0g; Protein: 6g; Potassium: 515mg; Magnesium: 99mg; Vitamin K: 2mcg

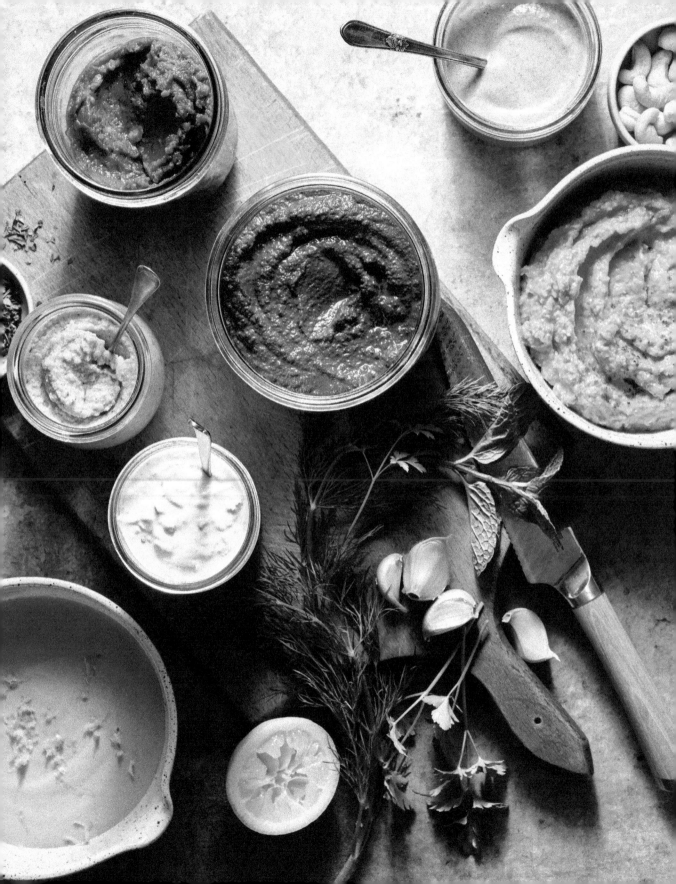

Sauces and Staples

Blueberry Chia Jelly

5 Ingredients or Fewer, Extra-Low Sodium, Gluten-Free, One-Pot
Serves 12 / Prep time: 10 minutes, plus 20 minutes to chill / Cook time: 5 minutes

This jelly goes well with pretty much everything. Its subtle flavor provides a perfect pop of vibrancy for both sweet and savory dishes—and adds significant health benefits. Chia seeds are incredible for heart health because they are high in soluble fiber, omega-3 fatty acids, and protein.

2 cups frozen blueberries

2 tablespoons chia seeds

2 to 3 teaspoons lemon juice (optional)

1. In a small saucepan, heat the blueberries over medium-low heat and mash, leaving some chunks as desired. Stir frequently for about 5 minutes.

2. Stir in the chia seeds. If desired, stir in the lemon juice. Remove from the heat and stir frequently for 5 minutes, or until the chia seeds swell slightly, beginning to create a gel. Transfer to a mason jar or other airtight container.

3. Let set up in the refrigerator for at least 20 minutes. Serve chilled. Store in the refrigerator for up to 1 week.

Flavor boost: Add 1 to 2 tablespoons of date paste, maple syrup, or your favorite sweetener or 2 to 3 drops of liquid stevia to give it that sweet jelly flavor. Vanilla extract is another great addition.

Per serving (2 tablespoons): Calories: 20; Total Fat: 0.5g; Saturated Fat: 0g; Cholesterol: 0mg; Sodium: 0mg; Carbohydrates: 4g; Fiber: 1g; Total Sugar: 2g; Added Sugar: 0g: Protein: 0g; Potassium: 7mg Magnesium: 7mg; Vitamin K: 12mcg

Apple-Cinnamon Sauce

30 Minutes or Less, Extra-Low Sodium, Gluten-Free, One-Pot
Makes 1½ cups / Prep time: 5 minutes

Turn everything you eat into apple pie with this sauce—oatmeal, sweet potatoes, even chickpeas, mashed tofu, or celery. You name it, and I've probably tried it with this sauce on top. And let me assure you, whatever it is, adding this sauce *does* make it taste better.

¾ cup unsweetened applesauce

¼ cup water

Juice of 1 lemon

¼ cup unsalted, unsweetened almond butter

2 teaspoons ground cinnamon

1 teaspoon liquid stevia

1 teaspoon vanilla extract

1. In a high-powered blender, combine the applesauce, water, lemon juice, almond butter, cinnamon, liquid stevia, and vanilla and blend for 2 minutes, or until well combined.

2. Store leftover sauce in an airtight container in the refrigerator for up to 1 week.

Substitute it: Don't have liquid stevia? Use Truvia, date paste, or maple syrup instead.

Per serving (2½ tablespoons): Calories: 50; Total Fat: 4g; Saturated Fat: 0g ; Cholesterol: 0mg; Sodium: 1mg; Carbohydrates: 4g; Fiber: 1g; Total Sugar: 2g; Added Sugar: 0g: Protein: 1g; Potassium: 68mg; Magnesium: 19mg; Vitamin K: 0mcg

Health-Nut Cacao Spread

5 Ingredients or Fewer, 30 Minutes or Less, Extra-Low Sodium, Gluten-Free
Makes 5½ cups / Prep time: 15 minutes / Cook time: 10 minutes

Store-bought Nutella is mostly processed sugar and palm oil, as well as fat-free milk, whey, and vanillin (an artificial flavor), but this alternative is just four minimally processed ingredients. After having this version, you may be surprised at how much you prefer it!

¾ cup pitted Medjool dates

1½ cups water

3 cups unsalted roasted hazelnuts

¼ cup cacao powder

1. In a saucepan, combine the dates and water, bring to a simmer, and cook for about 10 minutes.

2. Meanwhile, in a high-powered blender, blend the hazelnuts for 2 to 3 minutes, until they reach a flour-like consistency.

3. Add the dates with their soaking water and cacao to the blender. Blend for 2 minutes, or until completely smooth and creamy.

4. Transfer to an airtight container and store in the refrigerator for up to 1 week.

Make it easier: It is important to have a high-powered blender for this spread to come out really creamy.

Per serving (¼ cup): Calories: 137; Total Fat: 12g; Saturated Fat: 1g; Cholesterol: 0mg; Sodium: 0mg; Carbohydrates: 8g; Fiber: 3g; Total Sugar: 4g; Added Sugar: 0g; Protein: 3g; Potassium: 190mg; Magnesium: 34mg; Vitamin K: 3mcg

Three-Seed "Parmesan"

5 Ingredients or Fewer, 30 Minutes or Less, Extra-Low Sodium, Gluten-Free, One-Pot
Makes 2 cups / Prep time: 10 minutes

When a sodium-laden cheese can be replaced with a superfood
B vitamin boost, I can hear the hallelujah chorus. If you don't have this
homemade mixture on hand, in a pinch you can get a vegan parm—a
great one to buy is the shreddable wedge by Violife; it's available at
most grocery stores.

⅓ cup hemp seeds

⅓ cup raw pumpkin seeds

⅓ cup raw sunflower seeds

1 cup nutritional yeast

1 teaspoon garlic powder, or to taste

1. In a food processor, combine the hemp seeds, pumpkin seeds, sunflower seeds, nutritional yeast, and garlic powder and process for 30 seconds, or until it resembles a crumbly Parmesan cheese consistency, stopping and stirring occasionally to ensure it is well combined.

2. Transfer to an airtight container and store in the refrigerator for up to 2 weeks.

Substitute it: Instead of hemp, pumpkin, and sunflower seeds, feel free to use 1 cup of raw walnuts, Brazil nuts, pistachios, or whatever nut or seed you're craving. Also, if you'd like to add a pinch of salt, that's okay. It's better to add a pinch of salt to this nutritional powerhouse "cheese" made of seeds than to dislike it altogether and go back to the sodium-laden dairy option.

Per serving (2 tablespoons): Calories: 71; Total Fat: 4g; Saturated Fat: 0.5 g; Cholesterol: 0mg; Sodium: 11mg; Carbohydrates: 4g; Fiber: 2g; Total Sugar: 0g; Added Sugar: 0g; Protein: 5g; Potassium: 192mg; Magnesium: 47mg; Vitamin K: 0mcg

Herbed Chickpea Spread

30 Minutes or Less, Extra-Low Sodium, Gluten-Free, One-Pot
Makes 2½ cups / Prep time: 20 minutes

This spread may be healthier than herbed cheese, but it is absolutely just as flavorful, made from simple ingredients, and full of plant-based protein, iron, and fiber. Enjoy it as a salad topper, in a sandwich, or as a showstopper dip on any appetizer platter.

1 cup raw cashews

1 cup cooked or drained and rinsed canned chickpeas

¼ cup water, Save-the-Scraps Vegetable Stock (page 142), or store-bought low-sodium vegetable broth, plus more for blending

1 tablespoon fresh lemon juice

½ teaspoon garlic powder

½ teaspoon onion powder

½ teaspoon sweet white miso paste

2 tablespoons dried parsley

½ teaspoon dried dill

½ teaspoon paprika

1. In a food processor, process the cashews for 1 to 2 minutes, until they reach a flour-like consistency. Add the chickpeas and water and blend for another minute.

2. Add the lemon juice, garlic powder, onion powder, miso, parsley, dill, and paprika and blend for 1 to 2 more minutes, until smooth, adding more water or broth, 1 tablespoon at a time, as needed (up to 4 tablespoons) for a smooth consistency. Scrape down the sides frequently to ensure it is well combined.

3. Store in an airtight container in the refrigerator for up to 10 days.

Per serving (2 tablespoons): Calories: 48; Total Fat: 3g; Saturated Fat: 1g; Cholesterol: 0mg; Sodium: 22mg; Carbohydrates: 4g; Fiber: 1g; Total Sugar: 1g; Added Sugar: 0g; Protein: 2g; Potassium: 60mg; Magnesium: 22mg; Vitamin K: 5mcg

Tzatziki

5 Ingredients or Fewer, 30 Minutes or Less, Extra-Low Sodium, Gluten-Free, One-Pot
Makes 3½ cups / Prep time: 15 minutes

The only sauce more refreshing than this creamy, minty Tzatziki might be water itself! Put this healthified version of the Middle Eastern classic atop spicy curries, wraps, burgers, sandwiches, and even salad bowls or Mushroom and Bean Chili (page 54). I like Silk, Lavva, or Kite Hill brands for store-bought yogurt.

1 medium cucumber, grated

2 or 3 garlic cloves, minced

**2 cups plain plant-based yogurt,
store-bought or homemade (page 144)**

2 tablespoons minced fresh mint

½ lemon, juiced

1. In a large bowl, mix together the cucumber, garlic, yogurt, mint, and lemon juice until well combined. You can serve right away, but ideally, if you have time, put it in the refrigerator for about 20 minutes and serve chilled.

2. Store in an airtight container in the refrigerator for up to 1 week.

Flavor boost: Try fresh dill or parsley as well as, or instead of, mint.

Per serving (½ cup): Calories: 46; Total Fat: 1g; Saturated Fat: 0g; Cholesterol: 0mg; Sodium: 27mg; Carbohydrates: 6g; Fiber: 1g; Total Sugar: 2g; Added Sugar: 2g; Protein: 3g; Potassium: 146mg; Magnesium: 18mg; Vitamin K: 8mcg

BBQ Sauce

30 Minutes or Less, Extra-Low Sodium, Gluten-Free, One-Pot
Makes about 2 cups / Prep time: 15 minutes

This recipe is sweetened with potassium-packed dates and, to me, tastes better than store-bought sauce. It provides probiotic benefits from the fermented miso, glucose control from the apple cider vinegar, and antibacterial effects from the raw garlic. Use this sauce to marinate tofu and tempeh for sandwiches and wraps or on Hawaiian Pizzas (page 88).

8 pitted Medjool dates

2 or 3 garlic cloves, peeled

1 tablespoon coconut aminos or reduced-sodium tamari

2 teaspoons apple cider vinegar

Juice of ½ lemon

2 teaspoons sweet white miso

1 teaspoon onion powder

1 teaspoon salt-free chili powder

1 teaspoon smoked paprika

1 teaspoon ground cumin

¾ cup water

¼ cup chopped fresh tomatoes or no-salt-added tomato paste

1. In a high-powered blender, combine the dates, garlic, coconut aminos, vinegar, lemon juice, miso, onion powder, chili powder, paprika, cumin, water, and tomatoes and blend for 1 to 2 minutes, until completely smooth.

2. Transfer to an airtight container and store in the refrigerator for up to 1 week.

Substitute it: Instead of garlic cloves, try 4 teaspoons of garlic powder, and instead of smoked paprika, double the chili powder. Also, lemon juice and apple cider vinegar can be interchangeable if you have one but not the other.

Per serving (2½ tablespoons): Calories: 51; Total Fat: 0g; Saturated Fat: 0g; Cholesterol: 0mg; Sodium: 84mg; Carbohydrates: 13g; Fiber: 1g; Total Sugar: 11g; Added Sugar: 0g; Protein: 1g; Potassium: 138mg; Magnesium: 11mg; Vitamin K: 1mcg

Beet Spread

5 Ingredients or Fewer, 30 Minutes or Less, Extra-Low Sodium, Gluten-Free, One-Pot

Serves 8 / Prep time: 15 minutes

When I first tried my roommate, Elle's, beet hummus, I was inspired to make it again. While her version called for cooked beets and salt, we were both pleasantly surprised at how good this raw three-ingredient version tasted. We ended up elbow-deep in my Vitamix blender eating it straight with spoons, asking each other, "How is this so good?"

2 small to medium beets, peeled and cut into 1-inch cubes

½ cup tahini

Juice of 1 lemon

1. In a high-powered blender or food processor, combine the beets, tahini, and lemon juice and blend for 2 minutes, or until very smooth and creamy, stopping occasionally to scrape down the sides.

2. Serve right away or chill before serving. Store in the refrigerator in an airtight container for up to 1 week.

Flavor boost: Try cooking the beets first for a milder flavor. Make this sweet by blending in 4 pitted Medjool dates and ½ teaspoon of vanilla extract, or make it more like savory hummus by adding 1 can of drained no-salt-added chickpeas and 2 or 3 garlic cloves.

Per serving (2 tablespoons): Calories: 99; Total Fat: 8g; Saturated Fat: 1g; Cholesterol: 0mg; Sodium: 33mg; Carbohydrates: 6g; Fiber: 2g; Total Sugar: 2g; Added Sugar: 0g; Protein: 3g; Potassium: 135mg; Magnesium: 19mg; Vitamin K: 0mcg

Peanut Sauce

30 Minutes or Less, Extra-Low Sodium, Gluten-Free
Makes about 2½ cups / Prep time: 15 minutes

This sauce is a great accompaniment for fresh spring rolls, sushi, baked tofu, and simple grilled veggie kebabs. It is always a favorite.

1 cup packed pitted Medjool dates (20 to 25 dates, about 8 ounces)

⅔ cup simmering water

¾ cup unsalted, unsweetened peanut butter

Juice of 1 lemon or 1½ limes (about 3 tablespoons)

1 inch fresh ginger

1 garlic clove, peeled

Pinch red pepper flakes

1. Place the dates in a small bowl. Cover with the simmering water and let soak while preparing the other ingredients.

2. In a high-powered blender, combine the dates and their soaking water, peanut butter, lemon juice, ginger, garlic, and pepper flakes and blend for 2 to 3 minutes, until completely smooth and creamy. The sauce should be thick yet easily pourable. Adjust the spices to taste, adding more ginger, pepper flakes, and garlic, as needed.

3. Store in an airtight container in the refrigerator for up to 1 week.

Make it easier: To get the creamy consistency of this sauce requires a very high-quality blender. You do not want a chunky sauce! Also, the sauce will thicken as it cools and congeal in the refrigerator. Add more hot water as needed or if you prefer a thinner sauce when serving.

Flavor boost: Try adding coconut aminos or reduced-sodium tamari and orange juice to add more depth of flavor, or more garlic as desired.

Per serving (3½ tablespoons): Calories: 149; Total Fat: 8g; Saturated Fat: 1g; Cholesterol: 0mg; Sodium: 2mg; Carbohydrates: 18g; Fiber: 3g; Total Sugar: 14g; Added Sugar: 0g; Protein: 4g; Potassium: 243mg; Magnesium: 40mg; Vitamin K: 1mcg

Lemon-Tahini Dressing

5 Ingredients or Fewer, 30 Minutes or Less, Extra-Low Sodium, Gluten-Free, One-Pot
Makes 1½ cups / Prep time: 5 minutes

Salads can easily become overindulgent when they're drenched in dressings made with oils and sweeteners. Dressing doesn't have to be made with a laundry list of ingredients. Simply whisking together equal parts lemon juice (loaded with brightness and vitamin C) and tahini (which provides a grounding and subtle earthy creaminess and a great source of calcium and protein) is all you need to do to create this simple Mediterranean-inspired staple.

¾ cup fresh lemon juice (about 4 lemons)   **¾ cup tahini**

1. In a bowl, stir the lemon juice and tahini vigorously to combine. (Or blend in a high-powered blender for 1 minute, or until smooth.)

2. Transfer to an airtight container and store in the refrigerator for up to 2 weeks.

Flavor boost: I love this dressing plain and simple; however, it definitely doesn't hurt to add a little bit of garlic powder, ground cumin, paprika, or whatever spices and herbs you like.

Per serving (2 tablespoons): Calories: 93; Total Fat: 8g; Saturated Fat: 1g; Cholesterol: 0mg; Sodium: 17mg; Carbohydrates: 4g; Fiber: 1g; Total Sugar: 1g; Added Sugar: 0g; Protein: 3g; Potassium: 78mg; Magnesium: 15mg; Vitamin K: 0mcg

Save-the-Scraps Vegetable Stock

5 Ingredients or Fewer, Extra-Low Sodium, Gluten-Free, One-Pot
Makes about 8 cups / Prep time: 5 minutes / Cook time: 45 minutes

Instead of throwing away extra parsley, onion and garlic skins, or celery leaves and carrot tops, save them to make your own low-sodium vegetable stock. Place a large sealable container or zip-top bag in the freezer to put vegetable scraps in throughout the week. For this recipe, kombu (dried kelp) is included, providing a source of iodine, which is essential for thyroid function. You can find it in the Asian section in most grocery stores, in an Asian market, or online, or simply omit. Use this stock for the base of soups and when cooking rice or water-sautéing.

4 cups vegetable scraps

8 cups water

2 tablespoons apple cider vinegar

1 (10- to 12-inch) piece kombu

1. In a large pot, combine the vegetable scraps, water, vinegar, and kombu and bring to a boil. Reduce the heat to simmer and cook, stirring occasionally, for 30 to 45 minutes.

2. Using a slotted spoon, remove and discard any large scraps from the pot. Set a fine-mesh sieve over a large bowl and pour the broth through. (Discard the solids in the sieve.)

3. Transfer to airtight containers and allow to cool before sealing. Store in the refrigerator for up to 1 week or in the freezer for up to 3 months.

Flavor boost: Add whatever herbs and spices that you like, and even the sweet liquid from canned corn or the savory aquafaba from canned beans. Keep in mind that the taste and look of your stock will vary depending on what scraps you use. Beet tops, chard stems, red onion skin, and red cabbage will cause the stock to be slightly purple. Potato scraps will cause it to thicken. Cruciferous vegetables like cabbage and Brussels sprouts will make the broth bitter, so keep those to a minimum. Have fun experimenting!

Per serving (2 cups): Calories: 8; Total Fat: 0g; Saturated Fat: 0g; Cholesterol: 0mg; Sodium: 10mg; Carbohydrates: 1g; Fiber: 0g; Total Sugar: 0g; Added Sugar: 0g; Protein: 0g; Potassium: 20mg; Magnesium: 10mg; Vitamin K: 20mcg

Fresh Walnut Yogurt

5 Ingredients or Fewer, Extra-Low Sodium, Gluten-Free
Makes about 5 cups / Prep time: 16 to 28 hours

Think you need dairy milk to get the probiotic benefits of yogurt? Think again! Plant-based yogurt is a lot easier to make than most people realize. Don't be intimidated by the time it'll take to prepare. It's so easy and well worth the wait. You can find probiotic capsules online, from companies like LYFE Fuel (see Resources, page 150).

2 cups raw walnuts

¼ cup raisins

3 cups water, divided

1 tablespoon fresh lemon juice

3 multistrain probiotic capsules

1. In a medium bowl, cover the walnuts and raisins with 2 cups water and soak in the fridge overnight or for at least 8 hours. Drain and rinse.

2. In a high-powered blender or food processor, blend the walnuts, raisins, lemon juice, and the remaining 1 cup water for 2 minutes, or until completely smooth.

3. Transfer the mixture to a very clean resealable airtight container (preferably glass or ceramic) and empty the probiotic capsules into the mixture. Gently stir with a spoon or whisk until well combined. Cover with fine cheesecloth, muslin, or paper towel, and place a rubber band around the top to keep the covering in place.

4. Place in a warm area (75° to 80°F) for 8 to 16 hours. Transfer to the refrigerator to chill for at least 20 minutes.

5. Serve chilled. Store leftovers in an airtight container in the refrigerator for up to 1 week.

Substitute it: Instead of walnuts, try raw cashews, almonds, or Brazil nuts. Also try mixing 1 cup of raw walnuts and 1 cup of hemp seeds or raw pumpkin or sunflower seeds to get an even wider variety of fats, minerals, and antioxidants. Lastly, instead of ¼ cup of raisins, try 4 pitted Medjool dates.

Per serving (⅓ cup): Calories: 142; Total Fat: 13g; Saturated Fat: 1g; Cholesterol: 0mg; Sodium: 2mg; Carbohydrates: 6g; Fiber: 2g; Total Sugar: 3g; Added Sugar: 0g; Protein: 3g; Potassium: 118mg; Magnesium: 33mg; Vitamin K: 1mcg

Hemp Milk

5 Ingredients or Fewer, 30 Minutes or Less, Extra-Low Sodium, Gluten-Free, One-Pot
Makes about 3½ cups / Prep time: 5 minutes, plus 20 minutes to chill

Hemp seeds are an incredible source of omega-3 essential fats and essential minerals like zinc and magnesium, and they're packed with plant-based protein at 10 grams per 3-tablespoon serving. Plus, they're so cute and small they don't require a nut-milking bag! Hemp seeds blend up super creamy without needing to be strained, as with almond milk.

3 cups water

½ teaspoon vanilla extract

½ cup hemp seeds

2 pitted Medjool dates

1. In a high-powered blender, combine the water, vanilla, hemp seeds, and dates and blend for 2 minutes, or until smooth. Pour into an airtight container and place in the refrigerator to chill for 15 to 20 minutes

2. Serve chilled. Store in the refrigerator for up to 1 week. Shake well before using.

Flavor boost: Add 1 to 2 tablespoons of cacao powder for chocolate hemp milk.

Per serving (generous ¾ cup): Calories: 145; Total Fat: 10g; Saturated Fat: 1g; Cholesterol: 0mg; Sodium: 3mg; Carbohydrates: 11g; Fiber: 2g; Total Sugar: 8g; Added Sugar: 0g; Protein: 7g; Potassium: 324mg; Magnesium: 148mg; Vitamin K: 2mcg

Measurement Conversions

VOLUME EQUIVALENTS (LIQUID)

US STANDARD	US STANDARD (OUNCES)	METRIC (APPROXIMATE)
2 tablespoons	1 fl. oz.	30 mL
¼ cup	2 fl. oz.	60 mL
½ cup	4 fl. oz.	120 mL
1 cup	8 fl. oz.	240 mL
1½ cups	12 fl. oz.	355 mL
2 cups or 1 pint	16 fl. oz.	475 mL
4 cups or 1 quart	32 fl. oz.	1 L
1 gallon	128 fl. oz.	4 L

OVEN TEMPERATURES

FAHRENHEIT (F)	CELSIUS (C) (APPROXIMATE)
250°	120°
300°	150°
325°	165°
350°	180°
375°	190°
400°	200°
425°	220°
450°	230°

VOLUME EQUIVALENTS (DRY)

US STANDARD	METRIC (APPROXIMATE)
⅛ teaspoon	0.5 mL
¼ teaspoon	1 mL
½ teaspoon	2 mL
¾ teaspoon	4 mL
1 teaspoon	5 mL
1 tablespoon	15 mL
¼ cup	59 mL
⅓ cup	79 mL
½ cup	118 mL
⅔ cup	156 mL
¾ cup	177 mL
1 cup	235 mL
2 cups or 1 pint	475 mL
3 cups	700 mL
4 cups or 1 quart	1 L
½ gallon	2 L
1 gallon	4 L

WEIGHT EQUIVALENTS

US STANDARD	METRIC (APPROXIMATE)
½ ounce	15 g
1 ounce	30 g
2 ounces	60 g
4 ounces	115 g
8 ounces	225 g
12 ounces	340 g
16 ounces or 1 pound	455 g

Resources

Plant-Based Nutrition Information and Recipes

Cronometer nutrient analysis tracker

Cronometer.com

Cronometer is a nutrient analysis app that makes it easy to estimate your nutrient needs and track your food intake, as well as data such as your blood pressure, blood sugar levels, and heart rate.

Forks Over Knives website

ForksOverKnives.com

This website is an incredible resource for recipes based on the 2011 plant-based disease reversal documentary, *Forks Over Knives*, including a plant-based 101 beginners' guide, meal planning app, cooking course, and more.

NutritionFacts.org

NutritionFacts.org

Learn about the latest nutrition research through short video clips that make complicated concepts simple to understand.

Documentaries

Cowspiracy

Find out just how much our food systems impact the environment and our health. Cowspiracy.com

Forks Over Knives

Learn from plant-based medical professionals and hear relatable plant-based disease reversal transformations. ForksOverKnives.com

The Game Changers

Gain confidence in a plant-based diet and achieve optimal athletic performance. GameChangersMovie.com

May I Be Frank

Witness an incredible health transformation through plant-based nutrition, including holistic mindset and lifestyle changes. YourDailyVegan.com/portfolio-items/may-i-be-frank

Books

Barnard, Neal D., MD. *The Cheese Trap*. Grand Central (2017)

Buettner, Dan. *The Blue Zones*. National Geographic (2012)

Bulsiewicz, Will, MD. *Fiber Fueled*. Avery (2020)

Campbell, T. Colin, PhD. *Whole: Rethinking the Science of Nutrition*. BenBella Books (2013)

Cronise, Raymond, and Julieanna Hever, MS, RD. *The Healthspan Solution*. Alpha (2019)

Esselstyn, Caldwell B., MD. *Prevent and Reverse Heart Disease*. Avery (2008)

Fuhrman, Joel, MD. *The End of Heart Disease*. HarperOne (2016)

Greger, Michael, MD. *How Not to Die*. Flatiron Books (2015)

Hever, Julieanna, MS, RD. *Idiot's Guide to Plant-Based Nutrition*. Alpha (2018)

Ornish, Dean, MD. *Dr. Dean Ornish's Program for Reversing Heart Disease*. Ivy Books (1995)

Shopping for Plant-Based Ingredients

Imperfect Produce

ImperfectFoods.com

Imperfect Produce delivers a box of groceries that you pick weekly, including produce that wasn't aesthetically pleasing enough to be sold in grocery stores yet is still safe to eat to fight food waste.

LYFE Fuel

LYFEFuel.com

LYFE Fuel is a plant-based protein, algae omegas, and probiotic company that I am affiliated with. Use discount code "VITAMINKATIE" to save money when ordering the algae-derived DHA and EPA essential fatty acid supplement, as well as the probiotics needed to make Fresh Walnut Yogurt (page 144).

Misfits Market

MisfitsMarket.com

Misfits Market also allows you to build your own box of groceries and prevents food waste by utilizing produce from farmers that may be slightly aesthetically altered.

Rootly

RootlyShop.com

Rootly is a monthly subscription box filled with 12 new vegan grocery items. They also cater to allergies and other preferences and use plant-based, 100-percent curbside recyclable and compostable packaging.

Thrive Market

ThriveMarket.com

Thrive Market is a membership-based online grocery store providing organic brands at wholesale prices.

References

Akesson, A., C. Weismayer, P. Newby, et al. "Combined effect of low-risk dietary and lifestyle behaviors in primary prevention of myocardial infarction in women." *Archives of Internal Medicine*. Oct 22, 2007. 167(19): 2122–2127. PubMed.NCBI.NLM.NIH.gov/17954808.

Bailey, S., P. Winyard, A. Vanhatalo, et al. "Dietary nitrate supplementation reduces the O2 cost of low-intensity exercises and enhances tolerance to high-intensity exercise in humans." *Journal of Applied Physiology*. August 6, 2009. 107: 1144–1155.

Bonaccio, M., A. Castelnuovo, S. Costanzo, et al. "Ultra-processed food consumption is associated with increased risk of all-cause and cardiovascular mortality in the Moli-sani Study." *American Journal of Clinical Nutrition*. December 18, 2020. DOI.org/10.1093/ajcn/nqaa299.

Brighenti, F., L. Benini, D. Del Rio, et al. "Colonic fermentation of indigestible carbohydrates contributes to the second-meal effect." *American Journal of Clinical Nutrition*. April 2006. 83(4): 817–822. PubMed.NCBI.NLM.NIH.gov/16600933.

Chiuve, S., M. McCullough, F. Sacks, et al. "Healthy lifestyle factors in the primary prevention of coronary heart disease among men: benefits among users and nonusers of lipid-lowering and antihypertensive medications." *Circulation*. July 2006. 114(2): 160–167.

Dagfinn, A., E. Giovannucci, P. Boffetta, et al. "Fruit and vegetable intake and the risk of cardiovascular disease, total cancer, and all-cause mortality: A systematic review and dose response meta-analysis of prospective studies." *International Journal of Epidemiology*. February 22, 2017; 46(3):1029–1056. Accessed Wed. Oct. 21, 2020.

Danby, F. "Turning acne on/off via mTORC1." *Experimental Dermatology*. July 2013. 22(7): 505–506. PubMed.NCBI.NLM.NIH.gov/23800069.

D'Elia, L., G. Barba, F. Cappuccio, et al. "Potassium intake, stroke, and cardiovascular disease: A meta-analysis of prospective studies." *Journal of the American College of Cardiology*. March 8, 2011. 57(10): 1210–1219. PubMed.NCBI.NLM.NIH.gov/21371638.

Dickinson, K., P. Clifton, and J. Keogh. "A reduction of 3g/day from a usual 9g/day salt diet improves endothelial function and decreases endothelin-1 in a randomised cross over study in normotensive overweight and obese subjects." *Atherosclerosis*. March 2014. 233(1): 32–38. PubMed.NCBI.NLM.NIH.gov/24529119.

Erkkila, A., D. Herrington, D. Mozaffarian, et al. "Cereal fiber and whole-grain intake are associated with reduced progression of coronary-artery atherosclerosis in postmenopausal women with coronary heart disease." *American Heart Journal*. July 2005. 150(1): 94–101. PubMed.NCBI.NLM.NIH.gov/16084154.

Ferreira, L. F., and B. J. Behnke. "A toast to health and performance! Beetroot juice lowers blood pressure and the O2 cost of exercise." *Journal of Applied Physiology*. December 23, 2010. 110(3): 585–586. PubMed.NCBI.NLM.NIH.gov/21183624.

Gonzales, J., N. Barnard, D. Jenkins, et al. "Applying the precautionary principle to nutrition and cancer." *Journal of the American College of Nutrition*. May 28, 2014. 33(3): 239–246. PubMed.NCBI.NLM.NIH.gov/24870117.

Greger, M. "How to Lower Your Sodium-to-Potassium Ratio." *NutritionFacts.org*. August 11, 2020. NutritionFacts.org/2020/08/11/how-to-lower-your-sodium-to-potassium-ratio.

Gunnars, K. "6 Health Benefits of Apple Cider Vinegar, Backed by Science." *Healthline*. March 4, 2020. Healthline.com/nutrition/6-proven-health-benefits-of-apple-cider-vinegar.

Gupta, S., B. Sung, J. Kim, et al. "Multitargeting by turmeric, the golden spice: From kitchen to clinic." *Molecular Nutrition and Food Research*. September 2013. 57(9): 1510–1528. PubMed.NCBI.NLM.NIH.gov/22887802.

Hallberg, L., and L. Hulthen. "Prediction of dietary iron absorption: an algorithm for calculating absorption and bioavailability of dietary iron." *American Journal of Clinical Nutrition*. May 2000. 71 (5): 1147–1160. PubMed.NCBI.NLM.NIH.gov/10799377.

"Iodine." *National Institutes of Health Office of Dietary Supplements*. September 16, 2020. ODS.OD.NIH.gov/factsheets/Iodine-Health Professional.

Jennings, A., A. Welch, T. Spector, et al. "Intakes of anthocyanins and flavones are associated with biomarkers of insulin resistance and inflammation in women." *Journal of Nutrition*. February 2014. 144(2): 202–208.

Kelley, D., R. Rasooly, R. Jacob, et al. "Consumption of Bing sweet cherries lowers circulating concentrations of inflammation markers in healthy men and women." *Journal of Nutrition*. April 1, 2006. 136(4): 981–986.

Kjeldsen-Kragh, J. "Rheumatoid arthritis treated with vegetarian diets." *American Journal of Clinical Nutrition*. September 1999. 70 (3 Suppl): 594S–600S. PubMed.NCBI.NLM.NIH.gov/10479237.

Lucas, M., P. Chocano-Bedoya, M. Schulz, et al. "Inflammatory dietary pattern and risk of depression among women." *Brain, Behavior, and Immunity*. February 2014. 36:46–53. PubMed.NCBI.NLM.NIH.gov/24095894.

Orlich, M., P. Singh, J. Sabate, et al. "Vegetarian dietary patterns and mortality in Adventist Health Study 2." *Journal of the American Medical Association Internal Medicine*. July 8, 2013; 173(13): 1230–1238. Accessed Wed. Oct. 21, 2020.

Pes, G., F. Tolu, M. Dore, et al. "Male longevity in Sardinia: a review of historical sources supporting a causal link with dietary factors." *European Journal of Clinical Nutrition*. April 2015; 69(4): 411–418. Accessed Wed. Oct. 21, 2020.

Ras, R., J. Geleijnse, and E. Trautwein. "LDL-cholesterol-lowering effect of plant sterols and stanols across different dose ranges: a meta-analysis of randomized controlled studies." *British Journal of Nutrition*. July 28, 2014. 112(2): 214–219. PubMed.NCBI.NLM.NIH.gov/24780090.

Sacks, F. M., and E. H. Kass. "Low blood pressure in vegetarians: effects of specific foods and nutrients." *American Journal of Clinical Nutrition*. September 1988. 48(3 Suppl): 795–800. PubMed.NCBI.NLM.NIH.gov/3414588.

Satija, A., S. Bhupathiraju, D. Spiegelman, et al. "Healthful and unhealthful plant-based diets and the risk of coronary heart disease in U.S. adults." *Journal of the American College of Cardiology*. July 25, 2017; 70(4) 411–422. Accessed Wed. Oct. 21, 2020.

Vadder, F., E. Grasset, L. Holm, et al. "Gut microbiota regulates maturation of the adult enteric nervous system via enteric serotonin networks." *Proceedings of the National Academy of Sciences of the United States of America*. June 19, 2018. 115(25): 6458–6463. PubMed.NCBI.NLM.NIH.gov/29866843.

Willcox, D., G. Scapagnini, and B. Wilcox. "Healthy aging diets other than the Mediterranean: A focus on the Okinawan diet." *Mechanisms of Ageing and Development*. January 21, 2014. 136–137:148–162. NCBI.NLM.NIH.gov/pmc /articles/PMC5403516.

Wright, N., L. Wilson, M. Smith, et al. "The BROAD study: A randomised controlled trial using a whole food plant-based diet in the community for obesity, ischaemic heart disease or diabetes." *Journal of Nutrition and Diabetes*. March 20, 2017; 7(3): 256.

Index

About the Author

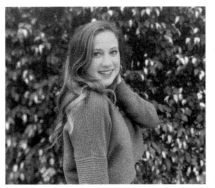

Katie Reines, MS, RD, also known as "Vitamin Katie," is a plant-based registered dietitian, certified vegan chef, yoga instructor, and food freedom and body image coach with a master's degree in human nutrition. As a plant-based foodie since January 2011, Katie taught her own series of vegan food demonstrations throughout college and was the head chef at retreats all over California and Hawaii. She also taught cooking classes for the patients at Dr. Fuhrman's Health Oasis in Boca Raton, Florida. Katie helps her clients make sustainable changes to transition to a plant-based diet through virtual one-on-one counseling, texting and voice memo accountability, personalized meal planning, and professional nutrient analyses. Her most popular program is "Feed Your Power," in which she helps women feed their bodies with healthy balanced meals as well as a mindset course to help them feed their minds from a place of empowerment, cultivating self-love and confidence.